from this moment ON

A GUIDE FOR

THOSE RECENTLY

from this moment ON

DIAGNOSED

WITH CANCER

ARLENE COTTER

MACMILLAN CANADA
TORONTO

Published in the United States by Random House, Inc., New York,
and simultaneously in Canada by Macmillan Canada, an imprint of CDG Books Canada Inc.

Acknowledgments and Permissions appear on pages 448–453

Library of Congress Cataloguing in Publication Data

Cotter, Arlene
From this moment on: a guide for those recently diagnosed with cancer

ISBN 0-7715-7640-4

1. Cancer.   2. Cancer—Patients.   3. Cancer—Psychological aspects.   I. Title.

RC263.C66   1999   616.99'4   C99-931421-1

This book is available at special discounts for bulk purchases by your group or
organization for sales promotions, premiums, fundraising and seminars. For details,
contact: CDG Books Canada Inc., 99 Yorkville Avenue, Suite 400, Toronto, ON, M5R 3K5.

Book Design by Arlene Cotter / abcotter@home   Final Composition: Stellar Graphics Ltd.

1 2 3 4 5 RH 03 02 01 00 99

We acknowledge the financial support of the Government of Canada through the Book
Publishing Industry Development Program for our publishing activities.

IMPORTANT
The ideas and views expressed in this book are completely subjective and meant only
as a guide to encourage individual exploration. The views presented by the author
should be used only as a reference and should in no way substitute for consultation
and treatment by licensed medical practitioners and healthcare professionals.

YOU WILL FIND YOUR WAY.

WE ALL DO.

FOR MY DEAR FAMILY & FRIENDS

FRANCESCO SARTORI

IZOLDA KOVACS COTTER & JULIUS COTTER

KATHY BODELL & LINDA HOLMES

ALWAYS, JÜRGEN GROHNE

DR. JOSEPH CONNORS

AND THOSE RECENTLY DIAGNOSED

WITH CANCER

JOSEPH BIRO

ELIZABETH & ROSE MARY BRAUN

CAROL CROMPTON

LESLIE & GRACE CZOTTER

LENKE GARAY

ROLF GROHNE

IMOGENE HOLMES

DR. JAMES IRONSIDE

BRENDA JOWETT & ILSE KOESTER

KATHLEEN KOVACS

MIRIAM MACPHAIL

MARY MCGARRIGLE S.S.A.

JACQUELINE OSBORNE

PAT ROSS (EWING)

MARIA SCHRATZ

DORIS STEELE

GERARD VANDEGRIEND

CELEBRATING

DONALD HENDERSON RADCLIFFE

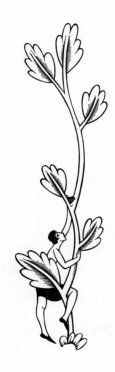

CONTENTS

A patient-to-patient introduction
to your cancer diagnosis that will help prepare
you for the challenging days ahead.

from this moment ON

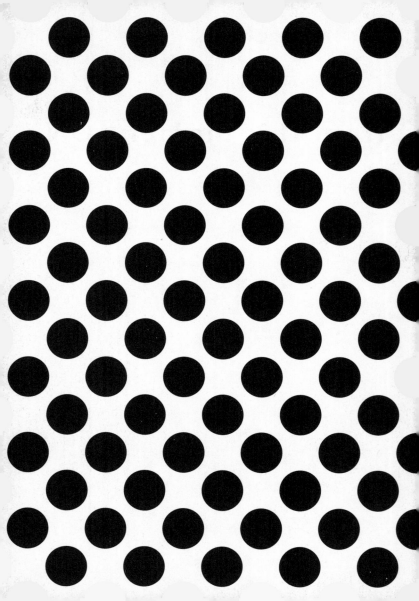

stop

Fortune favors the brave.

TERENCE

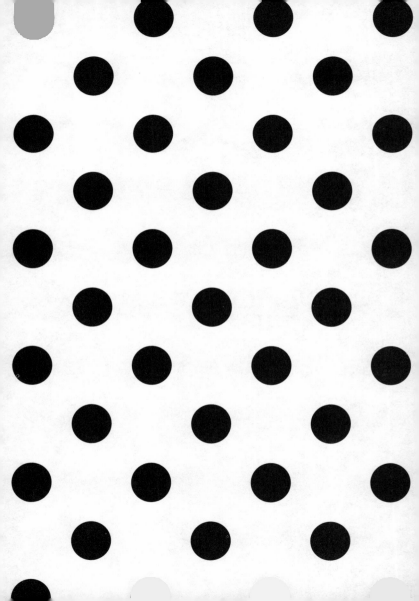

So, it's official.

You've been diagnosed

with cancer.

This time it's not some

family member,

acquaintance, or celebrity—

IT'S YOU.

Like it or not, you've joined

the cancer movement.

You're one of "them."

us People whose awareness
of our own mortality has been
irrevocably heightened.

More accurately, you're one of us.

And from this moment on...

your life will never be

the same.

Never.

Some things will be WORSE and
some things will be BETTER...

There will be many surprises
but also discoveries.

In the days ahead,
you will find YOUR OWN WAY
to deal with your cancer
diagnosis.

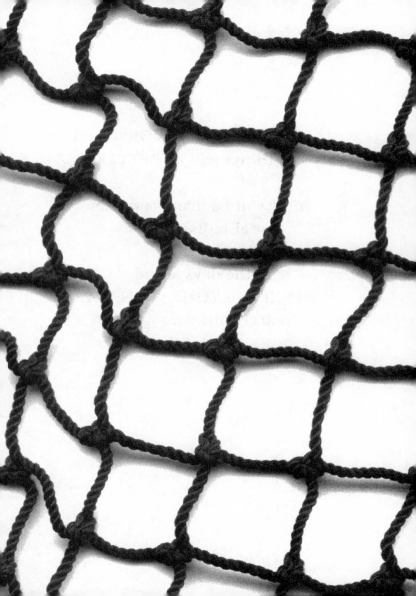

primer an introductory
book or text.
Oxford Concise Dictionary

Fortunately, with some PERSPECTIVE,
you can claim a measure of stability.

That's where this primer can help you.
It's a tool to guide you through
your initial cancer diagnosis because—
if you're like most people, you probably

don't know what to expect—

and that can be *terrifying*.

So take a good, deep breath and
create an opportunity to read quietly.
If you are unable to focus, ask someone
you trust to read to you.

Then, get ready for a **reality check**
because we're going to take stock
of the "situation"—together.

And the situation is this:

You have a life-threatening disease that requires your IMMEDIATE attention.

At this moment, there is NOTHING more important than stopping EVERYTHING else that you are doing in order to consider this.

Why?

Because understanding YOUR ROLE
in managing your own health
is the ONLY thing that
will allow you to

(continue to)

What does "quality of life" mean to you in *specific* terms?

_____

_____

_____

_____

live a life that has quality.

_____

_____

_____

_____

Think about it.
No matter how much others may
wish to help, you alone
must initiate the healing journey.

This is the first step.

Staircase drawing by Henricus Hondius, c. 1751

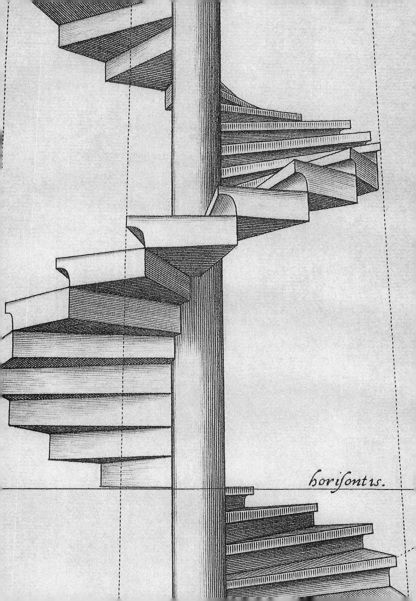

horisontis.

Whatever your prognosis,
you can prepare yourself
for the challenging days ahead
by accepting this fundamental truth:

It is completely within your control to
choose how you will respond
to the ways in which cancer is going
to change your life.

And it WILL change your life.

There will be a steep learning curve characterized by all the usual mistakes, setbacks, frustrations, and hard-won rewards of any worthwhile experience.

While it may SEEM obvious, sometimes you may need to remind yourself that:

You have the disease— the disease **does not** have you.

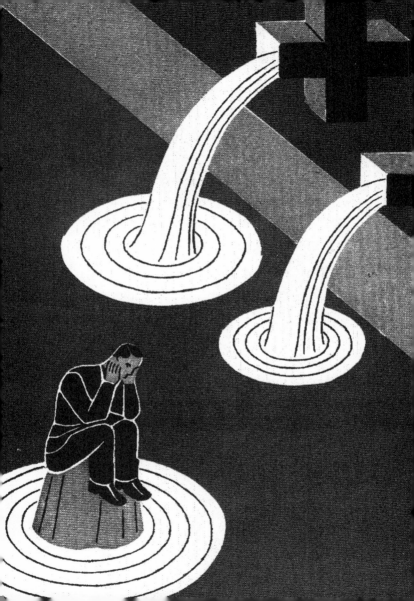

...everything can be taken from a man

but one thing: the last of human freedoms—

to choose one's attitude

in any given set of circumstances,

to choose one's own way.

— VICTOR FRANKL —

Man's Search for Meaning

Brian Cronin, *Man and Water Spouts* (detail), 1997
India ink and acrylic on paper, 17 × 18 cm
©Brian Cronin
This illustration first appeared in *The Atlantic Monthly*

You are a living, breathing, thinking HUMAN BEING and cancer is only an illness. You'll be amazed at how quickly you can wrestle back some power for yourself by

SAYING THESE WORDS

OUT LOUD:

"How I respond
to my cancer diagnosis
is my choice."

HOW I RESPOND

TO MY CANCER

DIAGNOSIS IS

MY CHOICE.

Try repeating this important message
every single day until it becomes a habit.

Go ahead.

Choose any response you're comfortable with. Cancer is an ordeal, but it is also an opportunity. *Exactly what kind of opportunity will be all up to you.*

Once you experience the benefits that come from GOOD CHOICES, you will instinctively start behaving in a manner

that will make things BETTER

for you—instead of WORSE.

This is an important time. WHAT YOU DO RIGHT NOW will chart the course for the rest of your journey.

That's why anything that helps you to feel better is a good idea. So, go ahead—*dare to visualize your own good health.* It will make the journey more bearable than projecting despair and gloom—even if you can only pull it off 5% of the time in the beginning. With practice and some discipline, you'll create a MAGNET for healthy thoughts, ideas, and encouragement.

No disease likes hope.

— HINDU PROVERB —

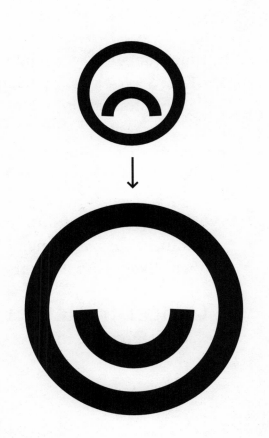

In time, cancer may become
the CATALYST for a very personal
transformation.

But many disturbing things
will likely happen to you first.

Everyone's experience is different,
of course, but over time,
you will likely pass through

A Cancer Initiation
something like this...

CANCER (*latin for crab*) is the fourth of the 12 zodiacal constellations in the visible annual path of the sun through the sky and identifies a person born when the sun is in its sign. The ancient Greeks discovered that the sun entered the constellation of Cancer at 23°27' North and thereby named the parallel latitude the Tropic of Cancer.

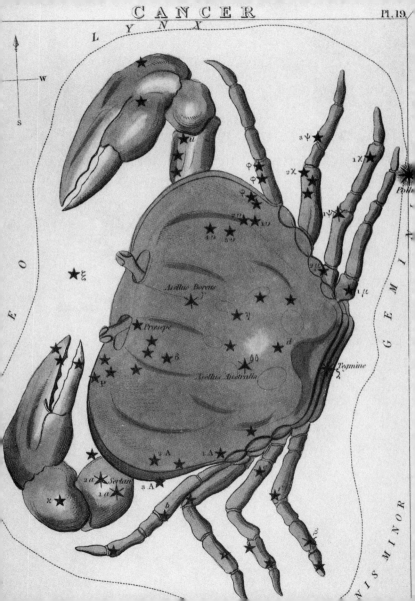

LYNX

LEO

GEMINI

CANIS MINOR

Asellus Boreus

Præsepe

Asellus Australis

Tegmine

Sextan

Pollu

From the time of diagnosis,

cancer will filter your perceptions
and responses—sometimes imperceptibly;
at other times, dramatically.

Significant life changes will occur.

You may feel

overwhelmed,

shocked, confused, devastated,
betrayed...and angry.

As the momentum builds,

daily life

may seem to slip from your control.

Soon your life may no longer feel like
your own. Things will start happening
around you—and quickly, too.

Probably faster than you can
realistically adjust to them.

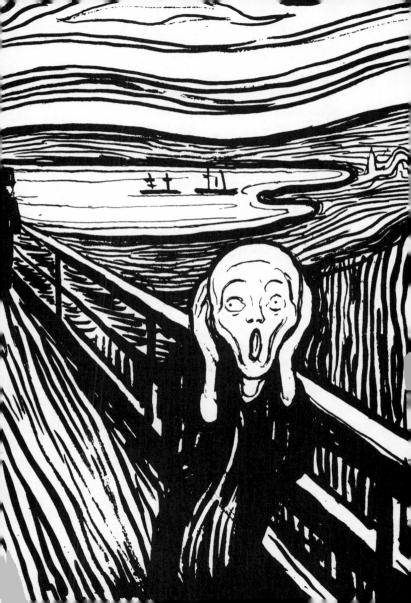

Likely, all the attention
coming your way from friends, family,
and healthcare professionals
will do much to sustain and distract you
during the INITIAL impact and panic.

Still, you may find that the physical
and emotional demands being made
of you are more than you can bear.

If your diagnosis is grave, *there
will be times of inconsolable
sadness, disappointment, and despair.*

grief deep or intense sorrow or mourning.
Oxford Concise Dictionary

There will be
grief.

"Grieving can't be hurried.

Grief will stay with you until you and your grief

are finished with **each** other."

MIRIAM MACPHAIL —cancer survivor and designer

*(And even then, it might
sometimes return.)*

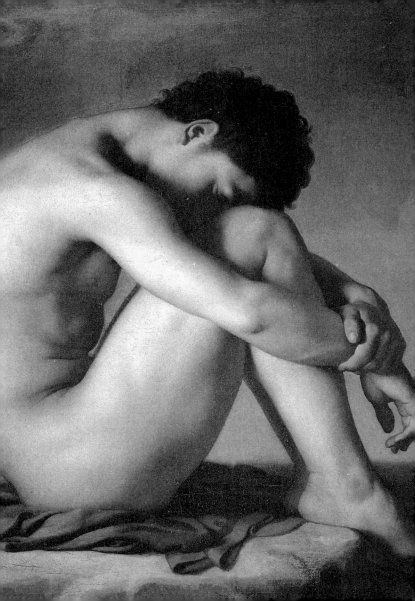

Grief is in itself a medicine.

— WILLIAM COWPER —

Charity

Hippolyte Flandrin (1809 – 1864) *Jeune Homme Nu* (detail), 1855
Oil on canvas, 98 × 124 cm
Musée du Louvre, Paris
Photograph: Erich Lessing / Art Resource, NY

In the beginning,
you may be desperate for

human contact

like companionship, hugs, and love.

Touch, care, and other acts of
loving kindness are immeasurable
and precious gifts to receive.

At some point, however, you're
going to need some

time alone

in order to examine your feelings
and gather your thoughts.

When you do, listen carefully
to the voices of your HEAD and HEART.

These intuitions are powerful guides for
your journey, and will see you through
all this *if you choose to listen to them.*

Some friends may react by
withdrawing from you because
they simply DON'T KNOW
what to do.

Of course, finding a quiet place
to examine your thoughts,
might be difficult with all the very real
DISTRACTIONS around you.

Likely, there will be a number of
diagnostic tests, appointments, and
interruptions to your solitude.

Your diagnosis will send a SHOCKWAVE
through those who know you. People who
are concerned might call or visit. Or they
may not, depending upon how they
react to your situation.

"As a caregiver you maybe feel more helpless

BECAUSE IT'S NOT HAPPENING TO YOU.

You're going through emotions on someone else's behalf.

You almost want to experience the physical pain

because all you have is this emotional pain—

and that's **invisible.**"

MAGGIE EDWARDS-PINEL

—caregiver to husband John, brain tumor survivor and professor

[TAKE ONE]

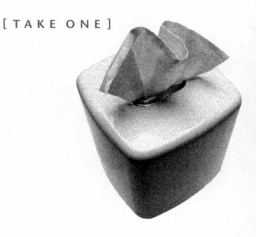

Friends and family will need time to adjust. They too, will be shocked. They too, will feel helpless. While you are trying to make sense of what has happened to you, so are they.

Besides their concern for you, and perhaps some inexperience in knowing what they can do to help you, YOUR cancer diagnosis is also reminding them of THEIR OWN MORTALITY.

Many people are uncomfortable THINKING, never mind TALKING, about their own death.

There's an elephant in the room.

We all know it is there.

We are thinking about the elephant

as we talk together.

It is constantly on our minds.

For, you see, it is a very big elephant.

It has hurt us all.

But we do not talk

about the elephant in the room.

— ATTRIBUTED TO TERRY KETTERING —

The Elephant in the Room

It can be hard trying to make sense of everything that is happening to you. For a time, you may be unable to do anything but simply accept the outpouring of energy, love, skill, and support offered to you by those caring for you.

You can gain much strength from people. However, at times they may not realize your FUNDAMENTAL NEED for quiet, rest, and sleep. When this happens, be polite but direct:

"I really need to rest now."

Odd as it may sound,

your confirmed cancer diagnosis could
be a HUGE RELIEF for you.

If you have been feeling unwell and
have worried for some time, it means that
steps can now be taken that will
help you to feel better.

Still, medical certainty comes with a
PRICE—loss of privacy. Your diagnosis will
make you the focus of activity and the
center of attention. Some of it will be
compassionate, some of it will be less so.

Kindness and professional care can be enormously comforting. All the personal attention is INVALUABLE for nurturing your health *but truthfully,* this focus on you and your needs won't last forever.

The IMMEDIATE crisis will pass.

One day all too soon,
your everyday concerns and patterns
of behavior will resurface—possibly before
you've fully come to terms with your
feelings regarding the diagnosis.

If your treatment or hospitalization
has been sudden, you may be distracted
by practical issues that take
IMMEDIATE priority over your personal
health concerns—

like major decisions regarding
family, business, work, school, medical
insurance, finances, child care,
and the host of responsibilities that
routinely govern your life.

diagnosis the identification of a patient's disease.
prognosis the forecast of the course of a disease.
Oxford Concise Dictionary

With all that's happening,
days may pass before you can
deal with all the demands,
and begin to consider your diagnosis,
prognosis, and treatment

options.

You may also find that, as practical
matters start to resolve themselves and
people's expectations of you
start to diminish, you'll experience
a more INTIMATE crisis.

There must be

This can't be

Why me?

I want to go back to

some mistake!

happening...

the way things were.

Please God, no...

When you're finally ready to accept it,
the full impact of your cancer diagnosis
will hit you hard.

REALLY HARD.

You'll be left to deal with the

reality

of what has happened to you, and
its potential consequences.

The Great Eclipse
The total solar eclipse shown here occurred near Guadalajara, Mexico, on July 11th 1991.
©CORBIS

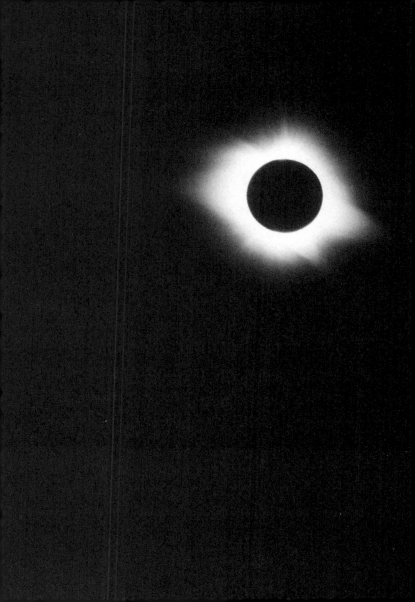

Lying awake at night,
you're certain to feel scared.

Some people feel they can best cope
by knowing as little as possible
about the disease.

They do this by dealing with each new
challenge as it presents itself—
never looking far enough ahead
to be overwhelmed.

This may be your standard coping strategy,
but it tends to work best only for those
challenges of an IMMEDIATE nature.

Dealing with chronic illness means
dealing with CONSTANT challenge.

This can be terribly stressful—

even more stressful
if you're not prepared.

What's worse than being unprepared,
is the fact that ignorance and avoidance
will ALMOST CERTAINLY harm you
in the long run.

You have some important
decisions
ahead of you.

The more you learn about cancer,
the better prepared you will be
to evaluate your options and make

GOOD DECISIONS
for your future.

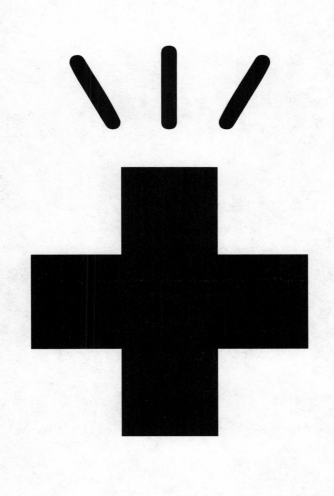

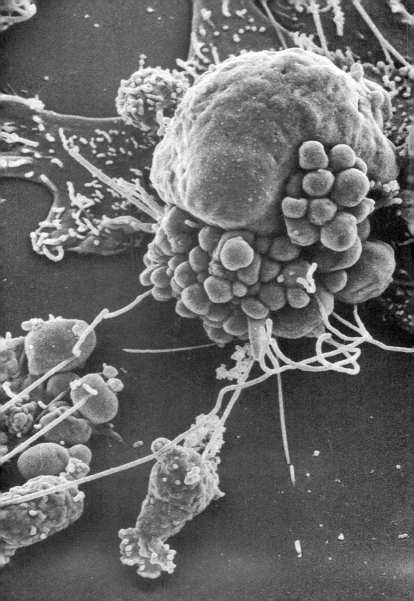

In this image, the large cancer cell LOOKS scary, but cancer cells are actually poorly developed and weak. The "killer cells" that surround it are powerful adversaries.

"You have cancer"

is one of the most feared medical diagnoses.

It's right up there with loss of sight, degenerative nerve and muscular disorders, brain damage, "flesh eating disease," and AIDS.

Our bodies have immune systems that defend our health every day by attacking mutant cells. Cancer cells like the large one shown here rarely survive an encounter with a healthy immune system's small but aggressive "killer cells."
©Boehringer Ingelheim International GmbH
Photograph: Lennart Nilson / Albert Bonniers Förlag AB

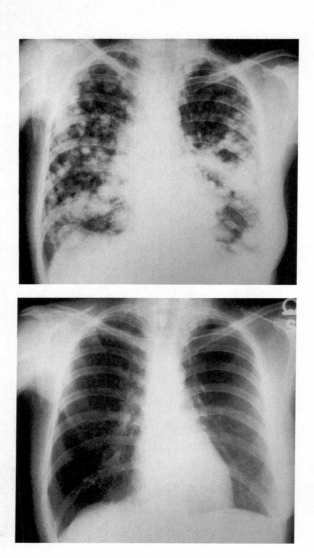

Technology allows us to view the
hidden regions of our bodies. This can
be terrifying because we can see the
tumors and the rogue cells that are
loose in our bodies.

Cancer is the general name
for many different chronic diseases,
all characterized by abnormal cells that
grow out of control and harm
normal tissue.

Some cancers are common, others rare,
some essentially harmless, and others...
life threatening.

Many cancers are fatal,
but some are not.

Chest X-rays showing the effect of hormone treatment for metastatic breast cancer. The
top X-ray shows numerous metastatic deposits of growing tumor throughout both lungs.
The patient was then treated by having her ovaries removed. This had the effect of removing
the natural source of estrogen hormone. Two months later, the metastases are gone.

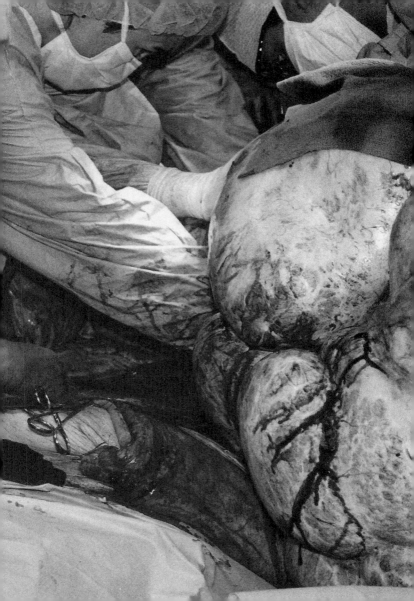

Sensational as it may be, this item in the *1996 Guinness Book of World Records* illustrates how incredibly resilient our bodies can be.

A rare case, the largest intact tumor ever removed was an ovarian tumor weighing 303.4 lbs. and measuring approximately 3 ft. in diameter.

The 1991 operation was performed by Dr. Kate O'Hanlan of STANFORD UNIVERSITY MEDICAL CENTER, USA. The 34-year-old woman made A FULL RECOVERY.

Photograph courtesy of Kate O'Hanlan, MD

Cancer frightens us because
we all know that there is still

no blanket cure.

This is hardly surprising since there are five major categories of cancer and over 150 different types.

ONLY WHEN you realize that each patient *(even those with the "same type" of cancer)* may or may not develop any one of a broad range of symptoms, that he or she might exhibit new symptoms, and that the time frame for disease progression in each individual often differs by many years, CAN YOU BEGIN TO APPRECIATE the enormity of the cancer field.

ill, you say?

Would that be...

acutely
chronically,
critically,
deathly,
fatally,
gravely,
mildly,
mortally,
seriously,
severely,
or...
terminally?!

Once you learn more about this complex
disease called cancer, you will appreciate
why it is unrealistic to expect BLACK and
WHITE answers from your physician.
There are just too many variables.

One refreshing antidote to answers
that are vague, indefinite, or unknown
is this medical reality:

There have been survivors of

every major type of cancer.

REMEMBER THIS FACT because
you may hear less encouraging words
in the coming days.

It's cancer!

I'm so sorry.

I'm going to do everything

Oh, my God!

You poor thing.

This is horrible.

How terrible for you.

What are you going to do?

Good Luck.

Good-bye.

I can to HELP you get well.

us

NEWLY DIAGNOSED patients soon discover that cancer has its own, well-defined vocabulary and culture.

Although your personal knowledge about the disease may be limited, most of us automatically associate cancer with another word for

MAXIMUM IMPACT—

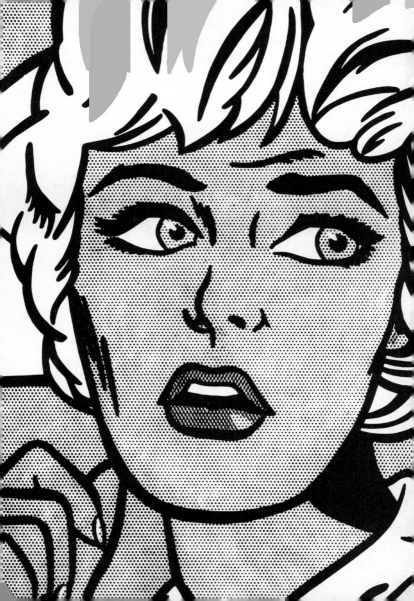

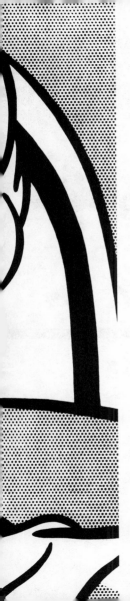

Roy Lichtenstein (1945 – 1997) *Nurse,* 1964
Oil and magna on canvas, 121.96 × 121.96 cm
©Estate of Roy Lichtenstein

vict

im.

i.e., "He's a cancer victim."

"Victim" may be a default choice
for your self-image when you don't
know HOW ELSE to handle what
is happening to you. Maybe weakness
becomes your only means of defense.

Being a victim is NOT a very powerful position.

It's NOT the sort of label that inspires a person with cancer to fight for his or her life!

Cancer "survival rate" is the medical term used to describe a specific period of complete remission. It varies, depending upon the type of cancer, generally from 5 to 7 years.

People have worked hard to overcome this cruel label.

The most-accepted jargon for those living through cancer is

cancer survivor.

You may prefer

survivor.

But—NOT... so... fast.

You haven't **chosen,** much less

earned, THAT designation yet.

Do you see yourself

as a victim OR

as a survivor?

Do you **need** to answer this question?

Maybe it is worth
considering.

You'll choose your own coping strategy at some point, but NOW may still be

too early.

Give yourself some time to process things and don't expect answers to come right away. Your feelings and ideas about cancer will develop and continue to change OVER TIME.

CHRONIC FEAR isn't healthy.
Identify your fears and try to overcome
them. Friends, patients, counselors,
social workers, therapists, clergy, or
your physician may be of help.

It may help you to acknowledge
some things that might otherwise
keep you in a suspended state of shock,
disbelief, denial, and ignorance.
Any ONE of which could effectively

paralyze you with fear.
Why cap my tooth...why take lessons...
why do anything at all?

Some of the manifestations of fear—like
DISBELIEF, and DENIAL—can play a
valuable role in your *immediate a*bility
to function. However, don't count on
either as a long term strategy.

While denial helps make the "impossible" possible for some individuals, *prolonged denial* could waste valuable time you may need to evaluate your options and initiate a treatment program.

With most cancers, the sooner that you begin treatment, the greater your chance for success.

Let's take a **closer look** at fear.

being a burden + financial ruin +
shame + isolation + pain + defeat +
death + physical limitation + loss of
control and dignity + dependency =

fear²

Fear takes many shapes, but for most
people with cancer...

one fear stands above

loud noise
darkness
spiders

the rest—

falling
needles
dogs
public speaking
open or closed spaces
bankruptcy
blindness
heights
impotence
abandonment
rejection
failure

I'll give you a definite maybe.

— SAMUEL GOLDWYN —

Just maybe you're going to **die** soon...

Just maybe **you won't die** for a long time yet.

Health practitioners will tell you that it is very difficult to predict a person's time of death accurately, and that, frankly, most people would rather not know anyway.

It seems that the *exact time* of death is influenced by an individual's **personal agenda,** as well as their physical condition.

WHATEVER the duration of your life,

you're still here

and you've got some living to do yet.

And just maybe "living" is going to
require some CONSCIOUS effort
on your part and a really, really

big effort.

And there's something else...

The next phase of your **life** is also
going to require a great deal of your

courage.

...courage is fear that has said its prayers...

— ANNE LAMOTT —

Travelling Mercies: Some Thought on Faith

So, brace yourself.

We're going to talk **specifically** about some of the things you may fear.

If we shed some light on the dark truths and half-truths you've heard about cancer, you can begin to deal with a reality that may be less frightening than some of YOUR IMAGINED DEMONS.

In other words, you can gain some

control.

The goal here is to fear less.

If you're like most of us, you'll need to learn some ways to help you do this.

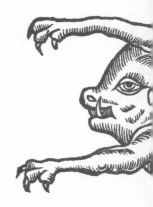

Sea creature sighted between Antibes and Nice in 1562
16th-century woodcut from Gesner's and Topsel's natural histories
From *Curious Woodcuts of Fanciful and Real Beasts* by Konrad Gesner
Courtesy of Dover Publications Inc., NY

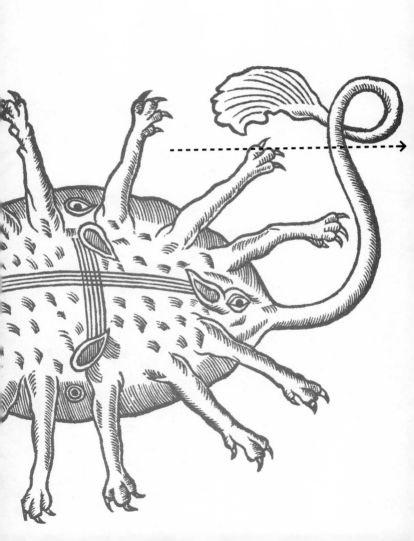

fearless=

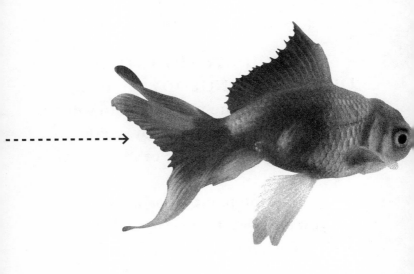

Fear. Less.

If you are doubtful
or cynical, NOBODY can hope to
explain to you the value of things like:
prayer, relaxation therapy, guided
imagery, support groups, or meditation.

At some point *(hopefully)*,
you'll decide to give something
a try, and, at that moment,

your world will get

much bigger.

Talk to people with cancer and cancer
survivors, and you'll discover what
kind of lifestyle choices are shared by
those people who enjoy a greater sense
of well-being.

Try this for yourself:

If you are afraid of some procedure—
like undergoing a bone marrow biopsy—
just ask along someone experienced in the
gentle art of therapeutic touch. They will
help to calm you and ensure that the
procedure is as painless as possible.

Ask around and you'll soon
discover many creative approaches that
patients use to overcome their fears and
improve their quality of life. *People will be
glad to tell you what has helped them.*

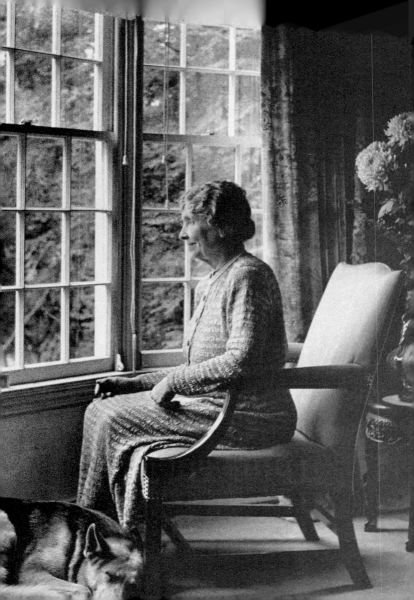

After fear, your next challenge will be

acceptance.

Yes, this is REALLY happening to you. *Complete* acceptance of your situation will occur by small measures.

Clearly, cancer will be less or more of a physical, psychological, and emotional violation depending upon your personal strength and values.

For your own sake, try to keep an open mind THROUGHOUT the journey.

Helen and Guide Dog Next to Window
Helen Adams Keller was an inspiration to generations of boys and girls, men and women, around the world. Deaf and blind from early childhood, this American writer and lecturer became a tireless pioneer for the rights of the deaf and blind.
Photograph: CORBIS / Bradley Smith

You'll come to realize that
there are no absolutes...

FACT

Two people receive the SAME treatment—
one has side effects...one doesn't...

FACT

Two people have the SAME prognosis—
one lives...one dies...

Many cancers are curable; others are considered to be
incurable. By lumping all types of cancer together, we arrive at
this dubious statistic: roughly 50% of those diagnosed with
cancer are going to become "survivors," and 50% will die.

Which person do you WANT to be?

It's true that you are one of many people with cancer, but you must never forget that you are an **individual** with a unique life—not a statistic.

If you still find yourself being drawn to the numbers, then try to be the "good" statistic.

Somebody has to be the good statistic... perhaps it will be you.

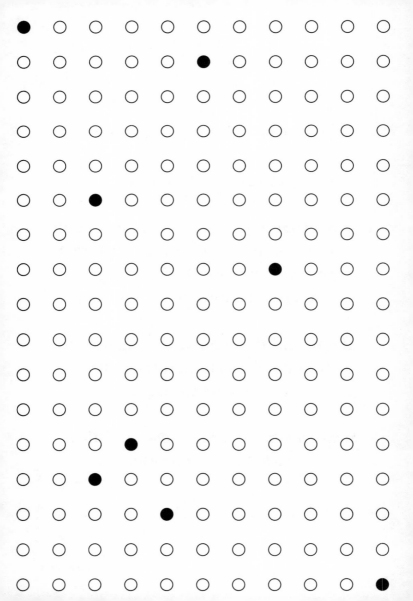

Think about it.

If you CONSCIOUSLY consider
what kind of patient you would like to be
and what sort of outcome you want,
then you can start to develop some goals.

You'll find it easier to **set goals**
for yourself NOW, before your mind and
body are further compromised by
symptoms and treatment.

Knowledge is power,

and you hold the balance of power here.

The fact is that **you** know more than anyone about yourself—important things like: how your body feels...the nature of your beliefs... the power of your will...and what you want to happen...

Or at least, you should know.

You may wish to ask your friend to
RECORD your answers to these
questions for review later.

If you're confused or uncertain about
some of these things, permit someone you
trust to ASK YOU THESE QUESTIONS
and listen carefully to your responses.

What is your body telling you?

**What beliefs do you have about
what has happened to you?**

How strong is your will?

What do you WANT to happen next?

(Your answers WILL change over time.)

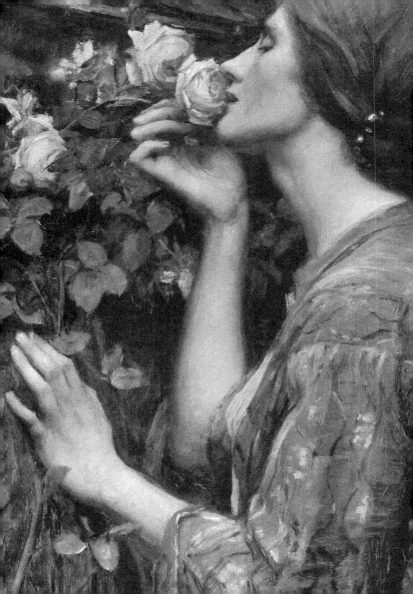

Consider these perceptive words.

It is much more important to know

what sort of patient has the disease

than what sort of disease

the patient has.

— SIR WILLIAM OSLER, MD —

Aphorisms

John William Waterhouse (1849–1917) *My Sweet Rose* (detail), 1908

It is NEVER wise to undergo any treatment that you don't feel has the potential to help you.

As an adult, *your life is your responsibility.*

Ultimately, it is YOU who will make the choices that will determine your specific course of treatment.

You may *even* choose to decline treatment altogether.

After investigating your OPTIONS, deciding against the recommended treatment is *always* an option.

While it is true that:

No one can eat for you...
No one can exercise for you...
No one can live for you...

More than likely, you'll *need* people
to help you get through this because your
ability to make sound decisions and to
take care of yourself may be

challenged by what happens NEXT.

Unfortunately, not all healthcare professionals treat every patient with kindness, dignity, and respect. Stories circulate of uncaring individuals and their actions. RUN from these people, and seek out those, instead, who are humane and compassionate.

You'll need a support team.

Things will be easier for you if you GENUINELY LIKE your team members and can form strong partnerships.

FOLLOW YOUR INSTINCTS.
Simplify your life by avoiding people who drain you of your energy. Instead, surround yourself only with those who contribute to your sense of well-being. You'll need their good energy, stimulation, prayers, encouragement, and support.

They'll need your trust.

I do not like thee, Doctor Fell.

The reason why, I cannot tell,

But this alone I know full well,

I do not like thee, Doctor Fell!

— MARCUS VALERIUS MARTIALIS —

Martial's Epigrams: Translation by Thomas Brown

Your own **health network** *(individuals who offer their professional and personal support)* will come together with time.

You can take the INITIATIVE by actively seeking out and selecting those who you feel are best qualified to help you.

You need not make the journey *alone*.

But you will need to take the first step.

Maurice Jassak *The Beckoning Forest*, 1995
Lynn Valley Park, North Vancouver, Canada
Color photograph
©Maurice Jassak

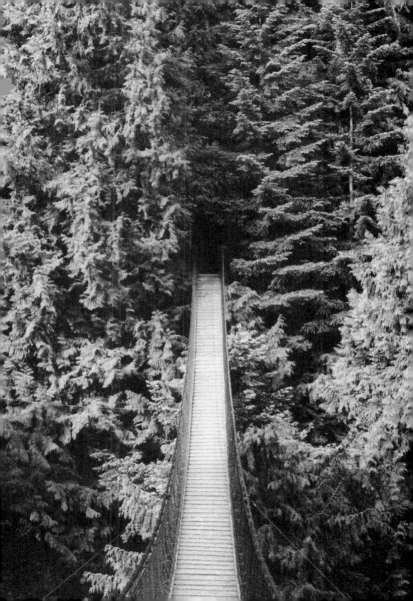

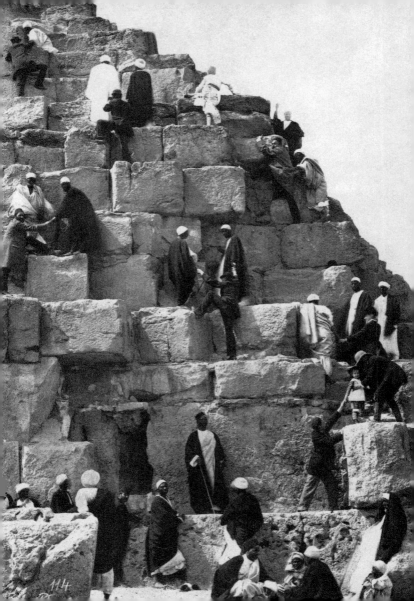

THERE IS NO EASY WAY
to speak honestly about what could
happen to you NEXT without facing
some disturbing possibilities.

The only consolation I can offer is this:

You are *not* the only person

with cancer.

And, you are *not* alone.

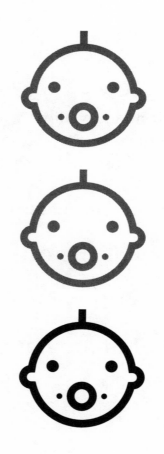

You, me, and *millions*

of people worldwide have

shared the cancer experience

in the past century.

Sadly, cancer has become a major
world health problem. Current medical
projections expect that

one in three

North Americans will develop cancer
in their lifetime.

abcotter@home *BabyFace,* 1995
Digital illustration
©1999 Arlene Cotter

Most of us diagnosed with cancer
in the Western world eventually find
ourselves in the care of oncologists
(cancer physicians) trained in
conventional Western medicine.

Other practitioners will likely participate
in your healthcare, depending upon
what type of cancer you have and how
your body is affected.

Your physician may seek opinions
from colleagues, or recommend
that you seek a second opinion
from an outside specialist.

If not, and you feel that more feedback would be valuable, request that other physicians also review your tests.

Because time is a CRITICAL FACTOR in the treatment of many cancers, you'll want to answer questions about your disease as soon as possible.

Traditional medical therapies initially tend to focus on the DISEASE by stopping the immediate growth of cancer cells, destroying existing tumor sites, and preventing the spread of cells to other sites (metastasis).

Western medicine currently utilizes three major treatment options, namely: SURGERY, CHEMOTHERAPY, and RADIATION.

Chances are that one or more of these treatments will be recommended to you. Medical science now recognizes some *additions* to these conventional treatments.

Emerging cancer therapies include immunotherapy or biological therapy—treatments like gene therapy, hormone therapy, vaccines, and bone marrow transplants.

Your medical team will provide an assessment and design a **treatment plan** specifically for you.

Usually your oncologist will schedule a formal information meeting for you and those people who are close to you. This provides an opportunity for everyone to ask questions and raise any concerns they might have regarding your treatment. You may choose to undergo some, if not all, of the treatments recommended to you by your healthcare team.

(Would you do it, Doc?)

Your treatment plan may include **curative** protocols aimed at managing your symptoms and eliminating cancer from within your body.

Where cure is not expected, due to the extent of disease and the limitations of therapy, **palliative** care strives to maintain your *quality of life*—by managing pain and symptoms, and by providing ongoing psychological and social support.

The treatments that you receive under these two headings are often identical. *The difference is the* GOAL *of the therapy.*

You and your

physician

will want to develop

your goals,

together.

Once called "alternative medicine,"
complementary therapies exist
*alongside conventional Western medicine
and are primarily concerned with stimulation
of the body's natural ability to heal itself.*

This is done using energy work, diet,
nutrition, vitamins, minerals and herbs,
exercise, and the development of the
mind-body techniques like biofeedback,
relaxation, visualization, and meditation.

In treating a patient, let your first thought be
to strengthen his natural vitality.

— RHASES —

Complementary therapies used to promote healing are TOO DIVERSE AND NUMEROUS to name here. They range from common practices like chiropractic to less conventional, but increasingly popular, approaches like naturopathy, therapeutic touch, homeopathy, macrobiotics, and aromatherapy.

Many traditional **Eastern** disciplines are accessible throughout the Western world including: qigong, acupuncture, and kundalini yoga. *Countless ethnic and folk remedies are also available for those who seek them.*

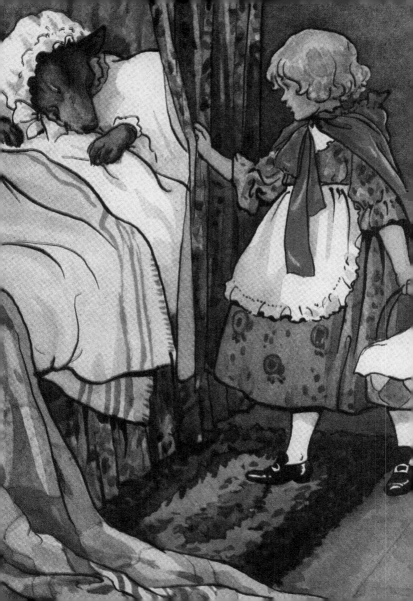

caveat emptor
the principle that the buyer alone
is responsible if dissatisfied; [Latin]
let the buyer beware.
Oxford Concise Dictionary

The discovery and CRITICAL evaluation
of complementary therapies will likely
become an ongoing exploration for you.
Remember this: desperate people can be
vulnerable—so, caveat emptor.
Be sure to exercise sound judgment.

Therapies that exist outside traditional
medicine are often unregulated, not
research-based, promoted by entrepreneurs,
and unrecognized by health insurance
plans. Ask patients and professionals for
referrals, recommendations, and opinions.
Collect as much information as you can
and only then—follow your INSTINCTS.

Illustration for *Red Riding Hood* by Margaret W. Tarrant, c. 1920

LITTLE RED: "Grandma, what great big ears you have!"
THE WOLF: "All the better to HEAR you with, Little Red Riding Hood!"

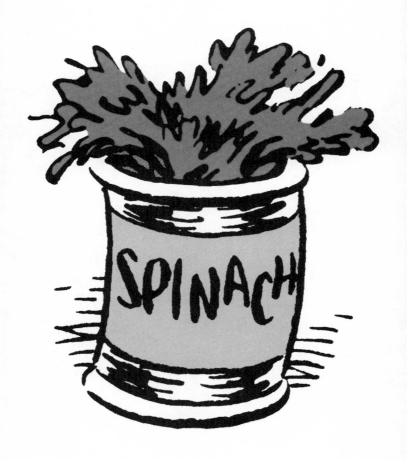

Many people who choose to undergo treatment for cancer incorporate BOTH traditional and complementary therapies into their **wellness plan.**

Clearly, the most logical treatment plan will acknowledge the need to **ARREST** the spread of the cancer, and to simultaneously **STIMULATE** your body's own natural ability to heal.

Both physical aspects are critical to regaining your health.

When seeking medical support,
remember the OBVIOUS:

Specialists
specialize.

Different members of your healthcare
team will make specific contributions. No
one individual can be expected to
address ALL ASPECTS of your care.

That's why, in addition to your oncologist and any other specialists, you will require the ongoing care of your family doctor.

Your doctor is best suited to consider the "whole person"—aspects of your OVERALL HEALTHCARE that may include referrals for nutrition, home care nursing, physiotherapy, pain and stress management, and psychological care.

If you are curious about investigative treatments and clinical trials, you'll want the added counsel of the practitioner who is *most familiar* with your lifestyle.

Take lists with you when you visit your doctor so that you are reminded exactly how you feel BETWEEN office visits. It is easy to forget specific facts that may help with your assessment.

It may surprise you
to realize that the focus of all this collective energy and skill is YOU.

As you become more familiar with the nature of your illness and the treatment options, you will likely assume a greater role in shaping your own healthcare program.

You'll find that the *more honest* you are about your feelings, and the *more clearly* that you communicate the facts of your condition, *the more likely it will be that you receive the kind of help you need.*

A bore is a man who, when
you ask him how he is, tells you.

— BERT LESTON TAYLOR —

There are times in life when this piece of
wisdom is simply NOT true. One of these
times is when you visit the doctor. You
probably have enough stress in life without
assuming the role of superpatient—
putting on a strong, heroic act for everyone and possibly neglecting *your real needs*.

AVOID second-guessing the meaning
of symptoms, censoring true feelings, and
trying to be "good." *Just be honest.*

What is the ALTERNATIVE to being
a "superpatient"?

Forget the cooperative, naïve, accepting,
accommodating, powerless, authority-
struck, helpless, and rather foolhardy "good
patient" stereotype of the past and
visualize yourself as someone

WHO TAKES AN

active role

IN YOUR OWN HEALING.

The **active patient** is the opposite of the patient who expects others (read: the Doctor) to shoulder the responsibility for his or her life.

An active patient may be strong-willed, curious, or demanding (and most likely is), but in order to qualify, must participate in his or her own treatment plan and healing.

After all, **if you don't care** about your own health, who should?

WHO WILL?!

What is realistically within your power will vary dramatically. Some days your energy will be average or perhaps even good. Other days, it will be NONEXISTENT.

Consider these guidelines:

1

It is part of the cure to wish to be cured.

— SENECA —

2

Take an active role in the development of your treatment and wellness plans.

3

Embrace the treatments in which you have faith and do everything WITHIN YOUR POWER to effect the best possible result.

People will assume
that you want to live and that you will
undergo treatment. Yet these issues are
NOT foregone conclusions.

They are important

decisions

that deserve your

ATTENTION.

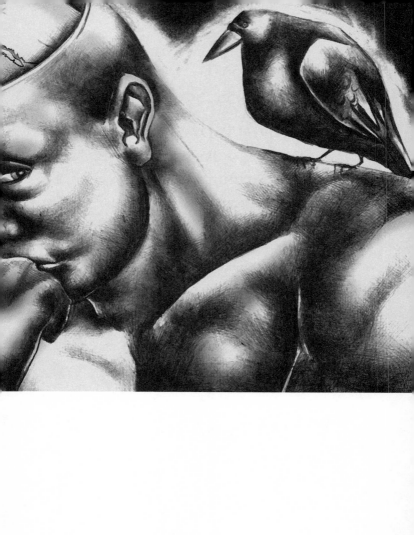

You could

choose conventional therapy.

You could

choose complementary therapy.

You could

choose a combination of conventional
and complementary therapies.

You could

forgo any and all forms of treatment.

*Let's explore some ideas that will
help you decide what to do.*

Patricia Leidl *Insight* (detail), 1995
Ballpoint pen on paper, 17.78 × 12.7 cm
©Patricia Leidl

Don't worry if you can't absorb these pages and all the information given to you right away—it's understandable.

YOU MAY EXPERIENCE
INFORMATION OVERLOAD.
You'll be bombarded with reading material regarding health issues. On top of this, stress and medication may compromise your ability to think and to remember. If possible, try to include another "set of ears" when you speak with your doctor or receive any kind of briefing. The objectivity, memory, and moral support of a friend *will be invaluable.*

There will be a lot of information to evaluate but as the days pass, your personal healthcare team and treatment plan will start to take shape.

As you become knowledgeable about your illness, and meet other cancer patients and healthcare professionals, you'll become familiar with the many

information resources like: libraries, the internet, public service agencies, treatment programs, clinics, financial aid, and support groups that are available within your local community.

Well-meaning folks will come forward with ideas, remedies, and articles in an effort to help you regain your health, or simply to show their support.

Some advice will be GOOD.

Some advice will be BAD.

While you may wish to hide from people—family, friends, peers, caregivers, social workers, healthcare professionals, mentors, therapists, spiritual counselors, whomever—they can provide the valuable ideas and experience that *you need to stay on track*.

It's a funny thing...

The people who you may have helped in the past are *not necessarily* the ones who will offer you their support. You may be astonished by the number of acquaintances and perfect strangers who will step forward in an effort to help

YOU GET WELL.

Although it may be very difficult for you to *allow* people to help you, once again—

LET THEM HELP!

As we review treatments
for cancer and the possible side effects
associated with traditional medical
interventions, remember that you may
experience NONE or SOME
of these things.

The intention is not to scare you but
to present a complete scenario of possibilities
that will help to prepare you for aggressive
cancer therapy should you require it.
And, should you choose to go ahead with it.

Prepare for the worst but hope for the best.

— ENGLISH PROVERB —

Here goes nothing...

Apart from the very real and very rare instances of SPONTANEOUS HEALING, remarkable and miraculous recoveries, without direct intervention, some cancers will inevitably spread and destroy your body's ability to function.

Depending upon what type of cancer you have and its stage of development, IMMEDIATE medical intervention may be critical in order to save your life. Shocking as it might be to hear, your doctor may want to commence treatment *right away*— as soon as he or she can schedule it.

If you decide to undergo traditional cancer treatment in order to stabilize your condition, your physician will likely recommend surgery, chemotherapy, radiation, or a combination of therapies.

These cancer treatments may terrify you. Cancer is an aggressive disease and these are aggressive measures. You've probably read that the SIDE EFFECTS of cancer therapy can cause you to feel even worse than your cancer SYMPTOMS.

This may be especially disturbing news if you are already experiencing discomfort or pain.

In an effort to arrest the growth and spread of cancer, organs, tissues, and even limbs may be **surgically** removed from your body. *Or not...*

Radiation (X-Ray, electron therapy, radium, cobalt treatment), **chemotherapy** (chemical or drug, hormone or biological treatment, and immunotherapy), or both, may precede an operation in an effort to first reduce the tumor size. Either or both of these therapies may be administered as a follow-up (adjuvant therapy), in order to (attempt to) destroy any remaining cancer cells. *Or not...*

Baldness can be more traumatic than the diagnosis for some patients because it shows vulnerability. If you go bald from your therapy, take it as a clear signal that the treatment is doing what it is *supposed to do.*

The possible side effects will
vary with treatment.

You may become frail, weak,
thin, moon-faced, burned from radiation,
bald, hairless, pale, covered with rashes;
or scarred from needles, biopsies,
and surgery. *Or not...*

Miriam MacPhail & abcotter@home *The Cancer People Series,* 1996
Digital illustration
©Miriam MacPhail and Arlene Cotter

There will likely be some uncomfortable

probing and poking

to your body

as you undergo a program of
diagnostic procedures including: blood
and urine analysis, imaging like X-rays,
computerized tomography (CT, CAT scans),
ultrasound, magnetic resonance imaging
(MRIs), or endoscopy (instruments
used for internal viewing of the body).
You may be prescribed a
confusing and complex assortment
(protocol) of drugs.

Time Out

*The following single page will offer you
a short and kind break from the harsh reality
of your cancer diagnosis, and all this talk
about possible treatments and side effects.*

*You'll find a little poem that's certain to
lighten your spirits, if only for a moment.
Please enjoy this brief and tiny magic
because after the poem, we will once again
return to disturbing subject matter—
just as abruptly as we left it.*

SNOWBALL

I made myself a snowball
As perfect as could be.
I thought I'd keep it as a pet
And let it sleep with me.
I made it some pajamas
And a pillow for its head.
Then last night it ran away,
But first—it wet the bed.

— SHEL SILVERSTEIN —

Falling Up

NOW...BACK TO WORK!
On top of this, you may experience
symptoms or side effects of lethargy,
chronic fatigue, pain, breathlessness,
constipation, diarrhea, nausea. *Or not...*

You could sweat profusely, have dry,
ruddy skin, no appetite, erratic bodily
functions, sores in your mouth, seizures,
delirium, or severe headaches. *Or not...*

At times, you may be unable to groom
yourself, find that you are prone to memory
interruptions and/or nanosecond
attention spans and apathy. *Or not...*

Most of the time when you do experience these symptoms, your healthcare team can assist you by reducing them, eliminating them, or, in extreme cases, by helping you to adapt to them.

Remember that patients undergoing radiation or chemotherapy are treated up to NORMAL tissue tolerance. In other words, you are given as much therapy as you can tolerate without destroying your body's natural ability to regenerate.

The balance between risk and benefit is *carefully* calculated for each patient.

During the course of your treatment,
it may be difficult for you to
DISTINGUISH between the side effects
of treatment and the symptoms of
your disease. For any number of reasons,
patients often (legitimately) associate the
treatment cycle with feeling awful.

One chemotherapy veteran, six
years in remission, chanced on her former
chemo nurse at a bus stop and threw up.

— WILLIAM MATTHEWS —

Dire Cure from *AFTER ALL: Last Poems by William Matthews*

What is happening

happening

I want to

I'm SO

to me?

feel normal.

tired of this.

"Two weeks later, I walked into the cancer agency—
not in my usual role as someone with a Ph.D.,
an appointment in the Faculty of Medicine, and nearly
30 years' experience as a healthcare professional—
but instead, as a 'breast cancer patient.'
This time, things were different.
This time, my confidence was GONE."

D R .   S U S A N   H A R R I S —cancer patient, professor, and dragon boater

"In essence, the male species with a male-only disease—
just as breast cancer is a female-owned disease*—had best
get over the mental disease endemic to men: **pride.**
Such is the protective male tendency to go into DENIAL
when there is anything involved in the nether
region below the belt, especially when involved with
sexual function, there is a blanket of silence."

ALLAN FOTHERINGHAM —cancer patient and journalist

Maclean's magazine

* Less than 1% of all breast cancers occur in men.

Throughout the ordeal, it will take enormous effort to STAY FOCUSED on

improving your health.

Sometimes you may feel so overwhelmed physically, mentally, emotionally, and spiritually that you find yourself with no energy and no will.

If you find yourself in this void, remind yourself that it may take 6 hours, or even 48 hours, to feel better. Ask for personal and PROFESSIONAL support to help you get through the bad times.

You may feel helpless to fight
the cumulative side effects of radiation
and/or chemotherapy for a time,
BUT THIS WILL PASS
sometime after the treatment ends.

If your treatment is aggressive, remind
yourself that this nightmare is a MEANS
TO AN END—an effort to ensure
your future well-being.

If you respond favorably to treatment,

there will be a **turning point**
when you will begin to feel better.

Realistic **goals** are important.

They will help you get through treatment.

It might help you to project a time of year, a celebration or event, planned for when this treatment cycle will be over.

* This doesn't mean to suggest that
you must be "up" all the time—that's
unrealistic and unnatural. It just
means that you want to AVOID the
slippery slope of giving up.

Encourage yourself often.

Find words or ideas that, through
repetition and force of habit, will keep
healthy thoughts uppermost in your
mind, and that will encourage you,
REGARDLESS OF JUST HOW BADLY
you might actually feel.

In the words of the wise—

*Fake it 'til you make it.**

I am reclaiming my strength.

— AFFIRMATION —

[YOU ARE HERE]

Illustration for *Jack the Giant Killer* by Margaret W. Tarrant, c. 1920

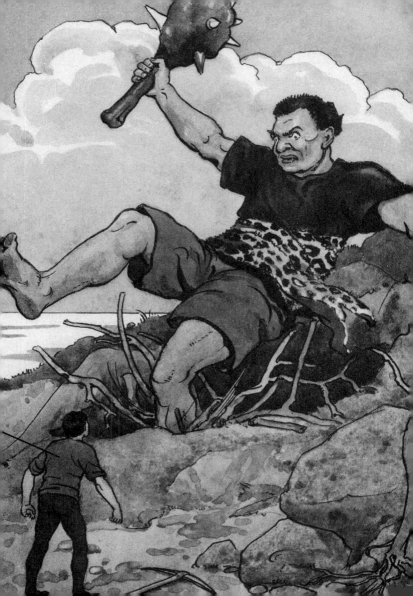

These famous words formed the biting inscription engraved on a golden ring. It offered a clever solution to the puzzling riddle quest: "What will make a rich man sad, and a poor man happy?"
King Solomon's Ring

This too shall pass.

— HEBREW FOLKTALE —

One day
soon
this will all be
behind me.

— AFFIRMATION —

Write down what you **need** or simply want to hear each day in order to feel better.

Share with your family and friends a list of things that they can say or do that will

encourage and inspire you.

Tap all your resources.

Hope, faith, and optimism
can exist alongside
common sense and logic.
Use them all to find your own way.

*Never rule out wishful thinking
and dreams.*

Here is the best part,

you have a head start.

If you are among

the very young at heart.

— YOUNG AT HEART —

Carolyn Leigh and Johnny Richards

As the days go by,
you may be surprised again and again
because—in between the periods
when you might FORGET—

you will REMEMBER that the
inconceivable has happened to you.

You have cancer.

Even "cancer veterans" experience
moments when they *just can't believe*
that they have cancer.

True, it's unfortunate

and disappointing that you have
been diagnosed with cancer. I don't know
ANY cancer patient who would wish
cancer upon someone else.

Perhaps it's surprising, too.

Maybe you have eaten well, enjoyed a regular exercise program, and done everything YOU COULD THINK OF in order to maintain a healthy body and balanced lifestyle.

Then again, maybe you haven't.

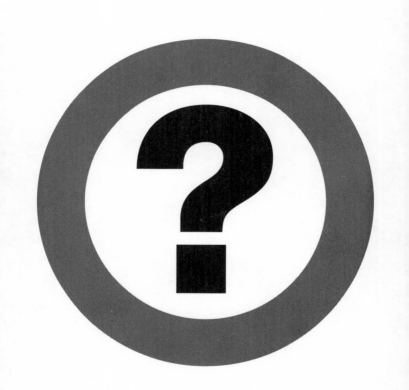

"Why me?"

Some cancers are **hereditary,** meaning that you are genetically predisposed to them. Others are linked to **lifestyle**— like smoking—and still others, to exposure to **environmental** factors like radioactive material.

Reading about cancer, you will find that not one but a NUMBER of factors have likely contributed to the onset of your disease. Some factors were within your control and others were *beyond it.*

Blame doesn't make you feel good about yourself and you NEED TO FEEL GOOD about yourself RIGHT NOW. Pat yourself on the back for making a start. Take it as a challenge to get your health back on track.

Cancer is indiscriminate. GOOD people get cancer, and so do BAD people. Don't get caught up in self-blame about a cause or causes that may or may not be relevant. Blame won't help you. But here's what might:

Choosing to live

your life well

from this moment on.

Look around you.

Think of ALL the people you've known—
people who are still living, and those
who have died.

Any amusing deaths lately?

— SIR MAURICE BOWRA —

heart disease
spinal cord injury
schizophrenia
dementia
Lou Gehrig's Disease
deafness
cystic fibrosis
addiction
multiple sclerosis
Parkinson's Disease
blindness
diabetes
muscular dystrophy
AIDS
leprosy
epilepsy
osteoporosis

(This is only a sampling of the human condition.)

"If you live long enough, you'll get something."

CAROL JORDAN —*the wise mother of*

Dr. Steve Jordan, oncologist and former medical director

Everyone has something
to confront in life.

And cancer is your SOMETHING.

Maybe cancer *is only one*
of the major challenges that you have
faced over the course of your lifetime.

Suffering is *universal,* so try not to feel as though **you alone** have been singled out to endure pain in this world. This realization may not make your grief less, but it WILL give you *some perspective.*

This is Catherine. I asked her to tell me her story and she did. *She told me that she is a painter and an art therapist. She told me that she loves to lose herself in the sea and in the sky and in the sunset. She told me that she will never tire of the moon and stars....*

What I had expected to hear was the story of her disability. What she told me was the evolving story of *her life.*

Life is *about* experience.
Each of us has our own unique and extraordinary story.

Nick Knight *Catherine Long for Dazed & Confused* (detail), 1998
Color photograph
©1999 Photograph: Nick Knight / Art Direction: Alexander McQueen

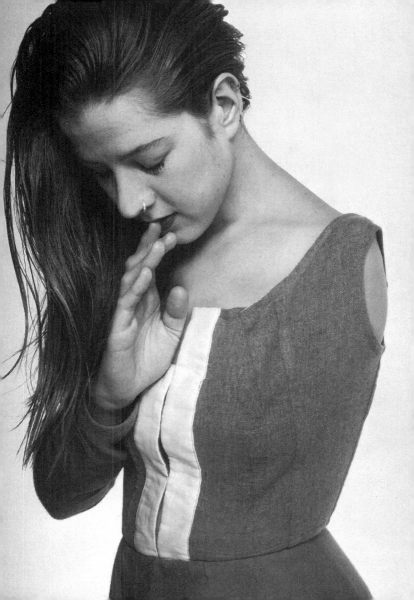

Nonetheless, not all experience *feels* that great.

It is HARD to cope
with life-threatening disease.

It is hard and it is stressful.

Stress

IS ONE OF THE MAJOR CHALLENGES that you'll have to face during your cancer diagnosis, and it is caused by all kinds of things.

Ironically, you won't have to search far to find medical studies that will confirm that stress likely contributed to the fact that your immune system is failing right now.

Nobody can argue the fact that too much stress can drain a person's energy. And, right now, you need all your energy to fight your cancer.

Perhaps friends and family can help reduce some of the pressure you may be feeling, if you can bring yourself to ask them for help.

Chances are that they will be grateful to be told *exactly* what they can do for you.

What things NORMALLY provide the physical, emotional, and spiritual energy you need to recharge your batteries and deal with stress in your life?

What about now?

While leisure activities like gardening, bridge, tennis, or fishing will likely be too demanding, you'll soon discover many healing activities that are more sedentary.

Things like reading, prayer, writing, meditation, music, visualization, yoga, and dreamwork can help *renew your spirit*.

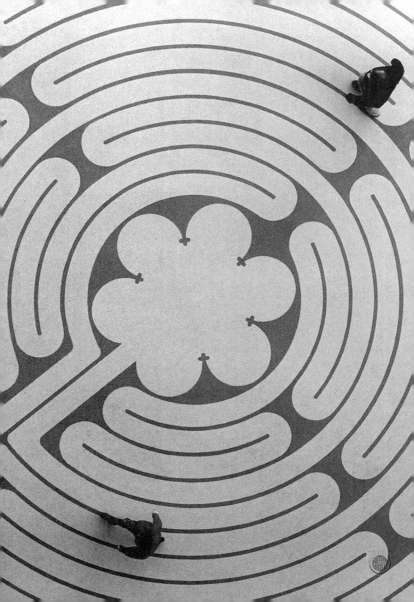

The LABYRINTH is one example of how multidisciplinary approaches to design and healthcare are helping to *redefine traditional healing environments.*

In 1997, San Francisco's CALIFORNIA PACIFIC MEDICAL CENTER and its *Institute for Health and Healing* developed this innovative environmental installation.

A 36-foot labyrinth—a walking mediation—now provides a popular and effective tool for those patients, medical center staff, and members of the surrounding community who are on their own *healing journey.*

Michael Macor *Untitled* (detail), 1997
Black and white photograph
The permanent labyrinth at the California Pacific Medical Center shown at 90° was created by *Stone Circle Design* and is based on the 12th-century floor design in Chartres Cathedral, France. ©1999 *San Francisco Chronicle* / Michael Macor

Healing takes time and energy.

Cancer is not just some stage of your life—it is a life-altering experience. It will take you some time to adjust to all the changes around you and inside of you.

Allow yourself to react naturally and honestly, always remembering the enormous well of PERSONAL POWER that we all have to draw upon.

Set your own pace.

Nobody is judging you, and judging yourself won't make you any healthier.

Try to be patient.

Whether slow or rapid, healing involves a
number of phases and lessons that require
physical EXPERIENCE and TIME,
not some intellectual shortcut.

Nothing quite compares with

experience. Not training, not education,
not instinct, not example. These things
may well prepare you, but you can't avoid
the pleasure and pain of experience.

In the days ahead, you're certain
to question much of what you THOUGHT
you *already* knew about life.

Let's discuss getting

THROUGH treatment.

You'll feel *less anxious* about
your cancer treatment
once you have an overview.

There are NO rules.

SOME avid skiers make weekly runs throughout the course of chemotherapy. There are those individuals who continue to work and manage their households during radiation, or soon after surgery. OTHER people take years to resume their regular activities. And some NEVER do. While many patients provide refreshing role models for resilience and spirit, sometimes a busy work schedule, financial pressure, or an ambitious exercise program could make difficult what might have been a more relaxed and *healing* recovery.

Try not to compare yourself
to other patients because
you simply can't know the specifics
of their situation.

We are all unique individuals.
Comparisons can be misleading and could
interfere with your own progress.

An imaginary ailment is worse than a disease.

— YIDDISH PROVERB —

Learn to "listen" to your own body
and make the decisions that
are best for you.

While treatment is different for everyone,
there are some universal experiences:

1

There will be **good** days and

there will be **bad** days.

Just like life.

2

The side effects

of radiation and/or

chemotherapy

are *cumulative*.

You'll be less able to "bounce back"
with each successive treatment.

3

In the beginning, you may start to feel
WORSE than you do now, due to the
side effects of aggressive treatment.
Be prepared for this.

If the program is successful,

ONE DAY YOU'LL START

TO FEEL BETTER—
thanks to the efficacy of these treatments,
and any complementary therapies that
support your healthcare objectives.

At the onset of treatment, it is natural that you'll want to keep participating in your usual daily activities. However, as treatment progresses, you may be unable to manage your responsibilities without some form of HELP.

Running errands may become unrealistic because driving a car, or even standing in a bus shelter, could require more physical energy than you can muster.

On LOW-ENERGY DAYS, you may need help to dress and feed yourself.

The physical limitations you experience may be difficult but

the psychological disruption

caused by cancer may be worse....

Prolonged anger signals that something's out of balance. Some hardy individuals use anger as a motivator and others direct it at people they know. Many turn their anger inward—a place where it is LESS LIKELY to be resolved.

There will be times of plummeting self-esteem,

fear

confusion

anger

grief, frustration, resentment, anxiety, and despair.

You used to be a person without cancer.
Now you're a person with cancer.

Your emotions may run wild. You might
experience an identity crisis—the difference between who you were BEFORE
all this happened and who you are
NOW that your ability to function
in your usual roles (parent, homemaker,
professional, worker, friend, lover,

whoever it was

that you were before this happened)

has been compromised.

NO MATTER HOW MUCH
SYMPATHY people offer you,
this is happening to you—
not to them.

You'll need to **accept** that your life is different—at least for now and perhaps from now on. You'll also need to make some big lifestyle adjustments.

You are different than you were.
You'll feel and possibly look different.
Your priorities will change.
You'll begin a much simpler life
that is out of step with busy people.

You'll be **different** from people who are healthy.

Accepting limitations and redefining yourself in relation to your CURRENT capabilities will help you to resist fear and depression.

You can't help but be changed
by life-threatening illness.
Losing control can be confusing
and frightening.

If you are sensible, you will learn to live
with your new limitations and try to
redefine yourself according to
your existing capabilities.

This will be an *ongoing* challenge for you
because what you are able, and not able,
to do will continue to change.

And, please remember this—

No matter what is happening
to your body...

the essence of

your spirit and personality

is still YOU.

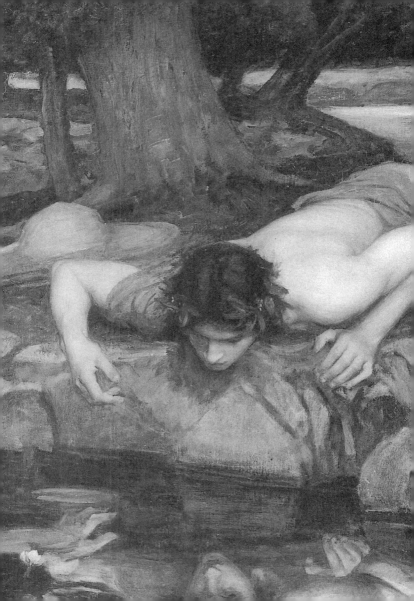

Make a conscious effort to assess
your own emotional and
psychological needs *from time to time.*
And when you do, try to be realistic and
compassionate with yourself.

Friends, family, and cancer support groups
can provide the invaluable feedback,
love, compassion, encouragement,

humor,

and stimulation that you'll need to cope.
You can do yourself a grave disservice
by "going it alone."

You are not your cancer;

yet you may have difficulty
RECOGNIZING yourself at times.

Don't be surprised if the size of your
world SHRINKS. It is understandable
that your new priorities will be basic.

Depending upon the extent of your
disease and the course of treatment,
for a time, your main activities may
be limited to eating, sleeping, bathing,
taking medications and supplements,
going for tests and appointments,
and undergoing therapy.

As simple as it sounds, simply
LOOKING AFTER YOURSELF IS
A FORMIDABLE CHALLENGE WHEN
YOU DON'T FEEL WELL.

Some of the time you'll feel
too sick,   weak,   impatient,
                                            restless or
foggy-headed to read,   watch TV,

sit at your computer, listen to the
radio or stereo, eat...brush your teeth, turn
over, talk

or even...smile.

Fighting for your health, and maybe
your life, will become a full-time job and
should be the FOCUS of your days.

Your health—

ultimately your life—

is what

everything

else depends upon.

It's an important agenda.

You may not be used to it, but you'll need to put your own needs first.

Some people always do, of course, but that's another story.

Your behaviors may change
(many times for the better)
but you must not lose your
"self" along the way.

The challenge to regain your health may
not be easy, so be charitable with yourself.

Forgive yourself again and
again—*as many times as you need to*—
because despite your best efforts to cope,
you may sometimes find yourself
acting in a manner that you don't like.

This is *perfectly normal.*
Like everyone else, you're entitled
to vent your frustrations.

"Perhaps the ONLY unforgivable act is not to forgive."

DR. MICHAEL HARLOS —*medical director palliative care, associate professor*

Any stress, discomfort, and pain that you experience may have a *really nasty effect* upon your moods. You may be cranky, self-focused, full of self-pity, and severely depressed. Sometimes you may wield your cancer as a weapon against others.

When emotions rage, remember that your cancer is affecting many people. EVERYONE is dealing with it as well as they can—*there are no scripts out there.*

Be good to yourself and also try and make *an effort* to be civil to those around you. This ordeal is difficult for EVERYONE.

Try to find a balance.
between focus and obsession.

It is easy to allow your mind to be
TOTALLY consumed with thoughts
of your cancer if you allow it.

Don't allow it.
You'll want to do everything you can
to help yourself heal, but you don't want
to subjugate the sum total of your life to
your role as *"a cancer person."*

PERIODIC withdrawal from people
may provide the time you need to
recharge your batteries, meditate,
listen to music, or just BE.

Make a special effort to stay in touch
with the world around you.

If you withdraw permanently, not only
will you become a cancer bore
(this is understandable and forgivable)

but you will have given

your own power AWAY.

At some point, your diagnosis
becomes something less
shocking to people.
IT HAS TO. They accept it.
They adjust.

OF COURSE, YOU MATTER.
Your life is important to you and to those
who care about you. Still, some days
it might seem bizarre to you that life's
banal activities go on *despite your own
poignant struggle.*

The kids still have to be picked up
from school, friends have to cut their
visits short for dental appointments,
to go to work, parties, concerts,
and shopping malls.

In other words, people keep on
living THEIR lives.

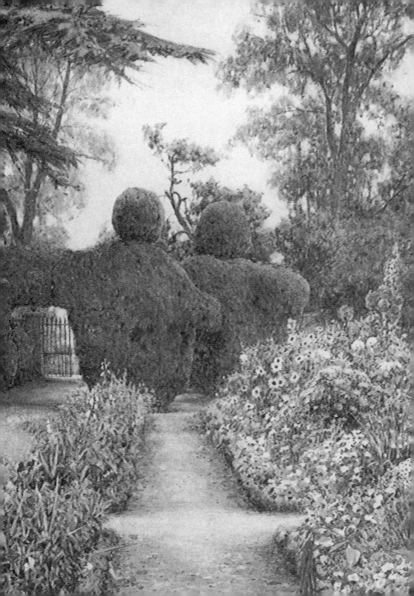

The world doesn't grind to a halt because you have cancer. Your situation may be life-threatening, and yet, as insensitive as it may seem at times, life goes on.

Sometimes you too will need A BREAK FROM EVERYTHING THAT HAS TO DO WITH CANCER. At these times, try and find something to do that will allow you to *forget all about "it."*

Do something **normal—** something that will make you happy.

Ernest Arthur Rowe (d. 1922) *The Gardens of Campsea Ash* (detail)
Watercolor, 30.5 × 47.5 cm
Private Collection

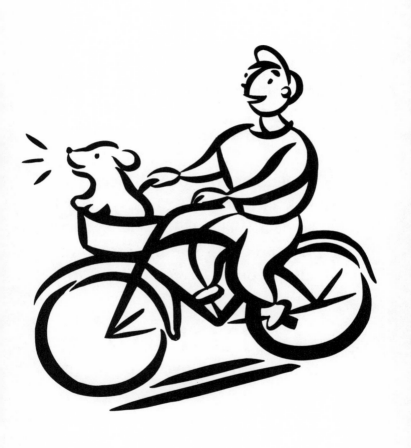

I CAN remember times in my life when I was *healthy* and happy.

— AFFIRMATION —

Laura Wallace *Boy on Bike*, c. 1991
Ink on mylar
©Laura Wallace
Courtesy of Canada Mortgage and Housing Corporation, Granville Island

THERE WILL COME A TIME
when you are ready to move on. You'll
come to accept your cancer diagnosis
as part—but not the whole—
of your life.

I'm sick of

being sick!

When this happens, you'll be ready
to start living *again*.

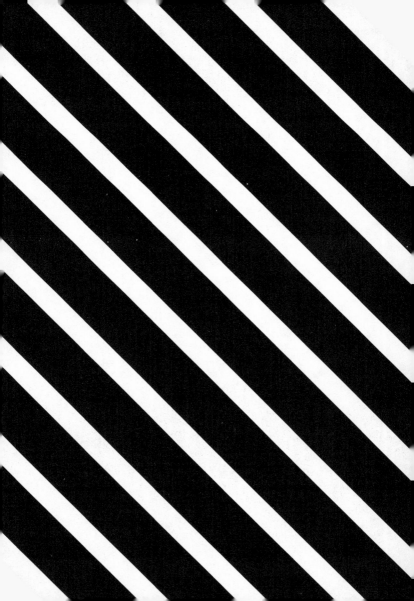

yield

He who has a why
to live for can bear with
almost any how.

FRIEDRICH NIETZSCHE

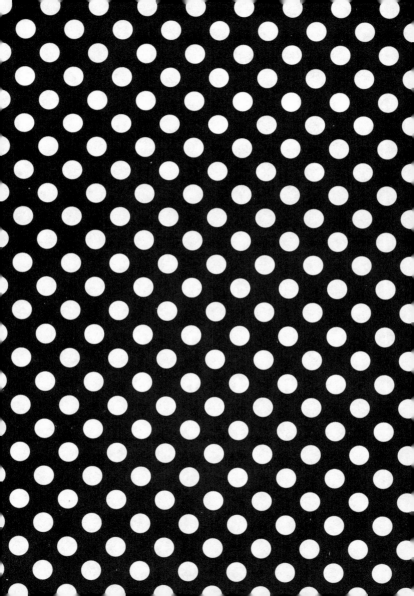

When *death knocks*
at your door,
it is a good time to

reconsider

your life.

Do you dare?

An oak and a reed were arguing about their strength.
When a strong wind came up, the reed avoided
being uprooted by bending and leaning
with the gusts of wind, but the oak stood firm
and was torn up by the roots.

— AESOP —

Aesop Without Morals translated by Lloyd Daly

You can **begin** here.

First, you should understand that
there is no right or wrong reaction to your
cancer diagnosis. You have your own
needs and personal style.
How you choose to deal with your
diagnosis is right for **you.**

Listen carefully to yourself
because your feelings are ALWAYS valid—
even if those feelings don't always
conform to other people's expectations.

After all, this is YOUR LIFE
we're talking about. Truthfully,
it is your own journey.

QUESTION

What does this ink blot represent?

ANSWER

Anything you want it to.

Linda Marie Holmes *Spot the Ink Blot,* 1999
Ink on vellum, 19.5 × 20 cm
©Linda Holmes

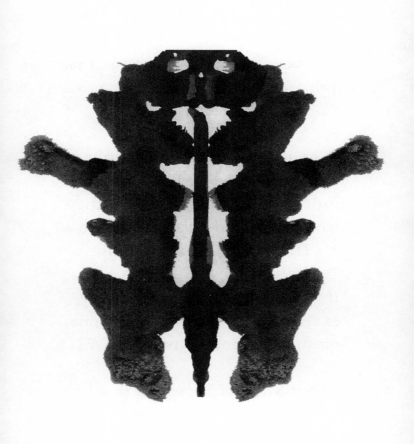

From your current perspective, it may surprise you to hear that cancer provides **several benefits.**

Challenge, confrontation, trying, failing, learning, *even suffering* are all aspects of a rich life. Remove these experiences, and you also remove all meaning from your life.

If you think this is nonsense, try to envision a life devoid of emotional, spiritual, and intellectual growth.

What KIND of life would that be?

The meaning of pain and suffering can be difficult, if not IMPOSSIBLE to understand. *Perhaps this will help.*

These are the words of a courageous young man who many of us watched— with mixed feelings of horror, compassion, and admiration—as he publicly battled cancer, during his Marathon of Hope.*

"The pain was there, but the pain didn't matter.

But that's all a lot of people could see; they couldn't see

the good that I was getting out of it myself."

TERRY FOX —cancer legend and international hero

---

*This remarkable story will be shared later in the book.

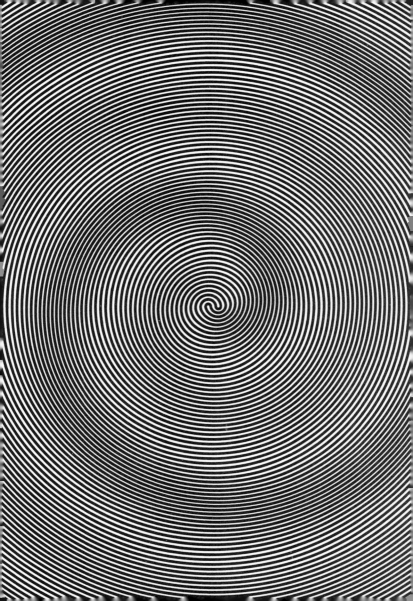

A Wake–up Call

Your daily routine is interrupted.
You are suddenly THROWN into
a state of hyper-awareness.

There are many ways to experience this intriguing pattern. One simple method is to stare
into the center of the image while you tilt the page from side to side.
From *Visual Illusions in Motion with Moiré Screens* by Craig Cassin
Courtesy of Dover Publications Inc, NY

WHO COULD KNOW?

After all I've done,
what **REALLY**
matters most to me
are my
relationships
with
loved ones.

Clarity of Vision

Since your time and energy
become so precious, you'll soon
discover WHO and WHAT is
fundamentally important to you

in your life.

THE ULTIMATE TRUMP CARD?

I'm
afraid that
I just
can't
eat my
peas
today!

Temporary Reprieve

This is a *legitimate* time-out from the busy world. For a brief space in time, ALL your external responsibilities will be lifted without question.

You'll be forgiven ALMOST anything.

I like all the special treatment, and feel **neglected** when people DON'T give it to me.

Lots of Attention

Energy, compassion, and prayers
will flow your way from
MANY SOURCES—including healthcare
professionals, friends, family,
caregivers, business associates, enemies,
acquaintances, *and even strangers.*

WHY NOT?

I've got
absolutely
NOTHING
to lose
and
everything
to gain.

A Second Chance

As your priorities change,
you'll have an opportunity to do
some things DIFFERENTLY
from now on.

If that's what you want.

I have **rediscovered** things about myself that I had LONG since forgotten.

Time for Yourself

Cancer isn't what most people
think of when they think of needing
some time to themselves.

But here it is—a big opportunity
for you to get to know your MIND and
your BODY *better than ever before.*

ONLY FOR THE DUBIOUS

If you're STILL not convinced that your cancer diagnosis could have its advantages, JUST FORGET ABOUT IT FOR NOW. Perhaps some other time you'll want to reconsider these very real and unexpected benefits.

Benefits or no benefits, living with cancer is an **ongoing process** of trial and error, of learning, and of relearning.

These RULES OF THE JOURNEY
will help you to cope:

1. Take it ONE step at a time.
2. DON'T be in a hurry.
3. Keep things really, really SIMPLE.

This is precisely how simple...

Do you want to

A Yes

B Only if...

C No

D Maybe

E I don't know...

live?

This is a BIG question and
there is a good chance that nobody
will ask you directly.

The assumption, of course,

is that you want to live.

THE OLD MAN AND DEATH

An old man once cut some wood and was walking

a long way carrying it. As he grew weary,

he put down his load and called Death to come.

When Death appeared and asked why

he had called for him, the old man said,

"To get you to take up my burden."

— AESOP —

Aesop Without Morals translated by Lloyd Daly

Allow yourself some quiet time
to focus on what is on your MIND and
what is in your HEART.

What do YOU have to live for?
Think about it and *only then*
answer from your heart.

Now, once again,

DO YOU WANT TO LIVE?

Perhaps the answer is clear and loud,
maybe it's qualified, or
perhaps you don't have one...yet.

And if you do,
even THAT may change.

Your head may be filled with
conflicting thoughts...

I want to live.

I demand a guarantee that I will get well.

Nothing can make any difference now.

I have nothing to live for.

My family needs me.

Who cares?

I still have things to do.

It's hopeless.

I don't want to deal with this.

I don't want to suffer.

What a relief.

I'll beat this thing.

"It's in God's hands."
"I'm leaving you."
"Don't abandon us."

"I need you."

"We can do this together."

Here is another question for you.

Given the challenges of life and
the absence of guarantees for your health
(especially if your prognosis is poor),

would it be **easier** for you to live

or

would it be **easier** for you to die?

For some of us, it's not the love of life but fear of death—nothingness, non-being, the unknown—that keeps us from dying. Sometimes it's simply the fear of being alone.

When we are healthy, we tend to forget how tenuous our life is, yet, deprived of oxygen for three minutes or water for five days, most of us will die.

But we usually WANT to keep on living.

When faced with a life-threatening situation, we are usually buoyed by an innate volition to live—even when our conscious mind is uncertain.

There are people who say they would
rather let themselves die, or even kill
themselves, than face terminal
illness. It is more common to hear
this from people PRIOR to diagnosis—
ATTITUDES CAN AND DO CHANGE
dramatically when time is finite.

Maybe the choice to fight for your life
comes quickly and naturally to you.
Maybe not.

If you CONSCIOUSLY EXPLORE your
feelings, you may surprise yourself.

The decision to fight for your life is
NOT a foregone conclusion for everyone.
Every person facing his or her mortality
has an opinion about which option would
present the greater challenge:

living or dying.

There are people who live full, rich, meaningful lives in spite of terminal illness. They accept that THIS IS THEIR LIFE JUST THE WAY IT IS, and they are grateful for the precious time allotted to them.

Faced with a very poor prognosis, you might conclude that dying would be easier for you than trying to live. After all, you have to do less. Much less.

In fact, doing

absolutely nothing

could really speed things up.

If you are physically weak, maybe you feel that rallying is well beyond your physical and mental potential.

You could be right.

Perhaps you'll choose to "roll over and face the wall" from here on.

Passivity is a powerful tool that can allow you to quietly accept your "FATE" without much of a fight for your life.

"GIVING UP" seems to set in motion all sorts of events that can bring death closer.

This is how it happens:

You consciously or unconsciously withdraw from the world, despite the
efforts of those around you to include
and stimulate you.

Withdrawal is a common
and merciful coping behavior, especially
when you're critically ill and DEPRESSED.

"Keep Breathing.

You Never Know When Life May Be Worth Living Again."

— ANONYMOUS GRAFFITI WRITER —

Off the Wall: Graffiti For the Soul

You may have good reasons for it, too.

I don't want to bother anyone.

They'll see me as weak.

They'll write me off.

I don't know what else to do, so I'll hide.

I need time to think.

I'll hide and return triumphant.

I'm not ready to talk about this.

I just don't care.

I'm exhausted and need my energy.

This is a private time.

I don't want pity.

I'll be unemployable if they find out.

I'm a liability.

If I ignore it, it will go away.

I'm scared.

Nobody really cares.

I have nothing to live for.

I'm going to die, anyway…

If you say "NO!" OFTEN ENOUGH to people, and continue to cut yourself off, naturally they will begin to relax their efforts, and include you less in their plans. And, after a while, they will go on with their lives *as though you no longer exist.*

If this happens to you, it is very easy to lose touch with earthly concerns and start to drift away from reality.

You could begin to feel that your life has become less important than the lives of others, because you are no longer a "REGULAR" (healthy) person.

M. C. Escher (1898 – 1972) *Symmetry Drawing A63 Pessimist-Optimist* (detail), 1944
Pencil and India ink, 18.2 × 28.4 cm
©1999 Cordon Art B.V.–Baarn–Holland. All rights reserved

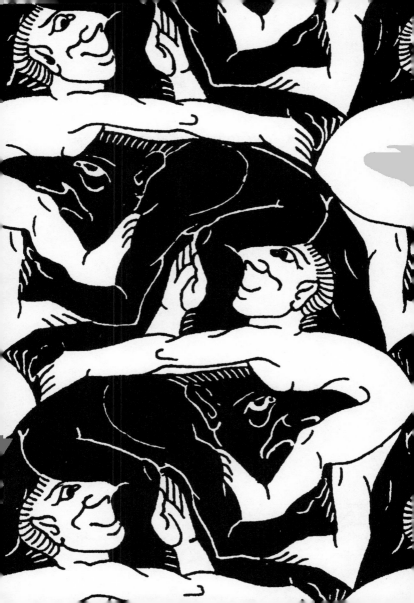

You may feel alone
and lonely.

It is such a secret place,

the land of tears.

— ANTOINE DE SAINT-EXUPÉRY —

The Little Prince

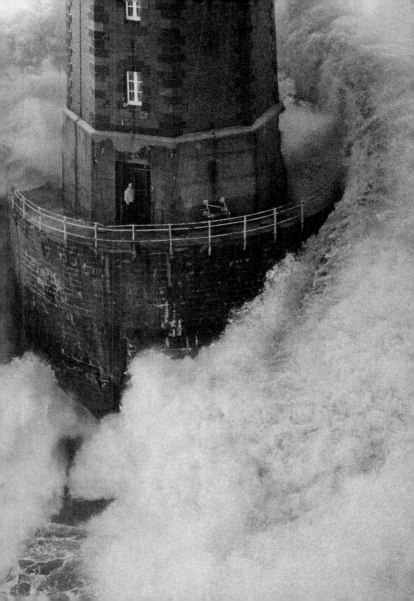

Stoicism the philosophy of the Stoics, a school of ancient Greek philosophy which sought virtue as the greatest good, and taught control of one's feeling and passions.
Oxford Concise Dictionary

It is reasonable that you might try to hold on tight to some measure of DIGNITY. So many of the things that are happening around you will be beyond your control. However, you "natural stoics" may want to consider the difference between

controlling your feelings
(which is healthy) and

repressing your feelings
(which is not so healthy).

Only lions

Stoicism is one reaction to your
cancer diagnosis that may suit
your personality but try to avoid
"martyrdom" as a full-time response.

like martyrs.

— UNKNOWN —

mortality the state of being subject to death; the inevitable cycle for life-forms.
Oxford Concise Dictionary

It is natural that you'll feel like giving up the struggle at times but if you make an effort, you can usually work through it over a period of days or weeks.

Exploring your own mortality might, but need not, lead to severe depression.

After all, mortality is a natural part of life—we ALL die sometime.

When asked about her longevity,
Jeanne-Louise Calment stated simply:
"God must have forgotten me."

It seems that He did not.

Jeanne-Louise Calment was **born**
in France on February 21st 1875.

The oldest authenticated human **lived**
happily for 122 years.

And THEN what happened?

She **died**—just like everyone else.

Do not try to live forever. You will not succeed.

— GEORGE BERNARD SHAW —

The Doctor's Dilemma

You'll need to talk honestly
about what you are feeling—
about living and dying—
with people who won't judge you.

Find someone you trust.

If loved ones find it difficult to accept
your thoughts about death without
feeling sad, angry, betrayed, or abandoned,
you may find it helpful to speak with
acquaintances in support groups, or
professionals who have YOUR
WELL-BEING at heart but won't be hurt
or frightened by your candor.

Admittedly, it's possible that once you inform yourself about your prognosis and examine your beliefs honestly, you might have a profound and lingering sense that your time is limited.

Perhaps you'll feel ready

to prepare for death. Many people have chosen this path.

I have done all that I was sent into the world to do, and I am ready to go.

— C. S. LEWIS —

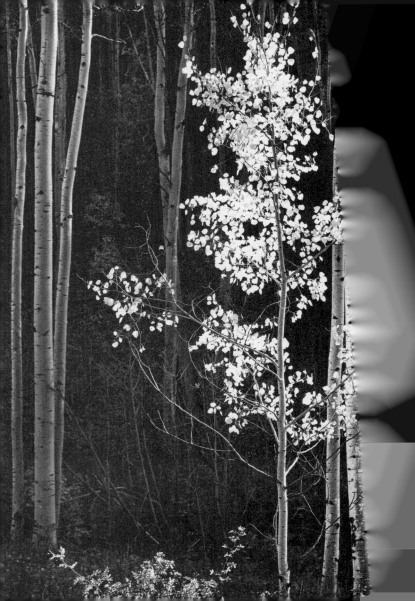

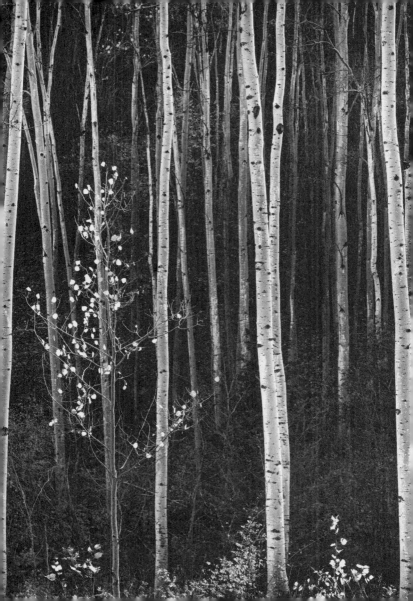

Most people will respect

your decision to give up the fight
and allow yourself to die—*sooner, rather
than later*—with relative dignity, before
this whole thing gets prolonged.

But probably not *everyone*.

Some people might *refuse* to let you go.

Energy sent your way through
the kindness, love, faith, prayers, hope,
and belief of others can do much to
sustain you during those times
when your own resources are depleted.
(You'll know it when you feel it.)

Yet, while optimism and faith are deep
and powerful allies for regaining health,
the core of WILL must come from
the person whose life is in jeopardy...

That would be YOU.

In order to have a good chance,
you have to want to live.

And if you don't want to live...

Ron Sangha *Burning Candles*, c. 1994
Color photograph
Original Art Direction: Kiky Kambylis / Letterbox
©Ron Sangha / Tony Stone Images, Vancouver

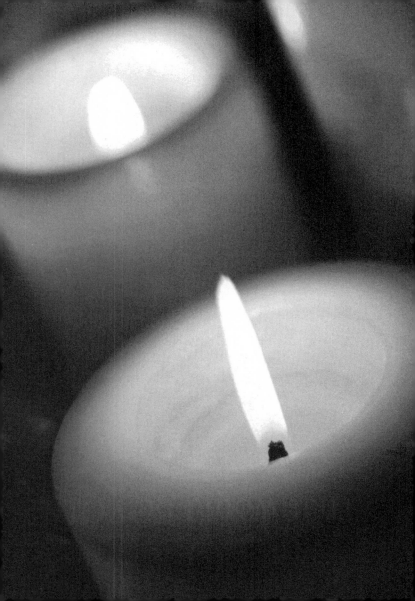

You can always choose
to let go.

No one can give you better advice
than yourself.

— CICERO —

Ad Atticum

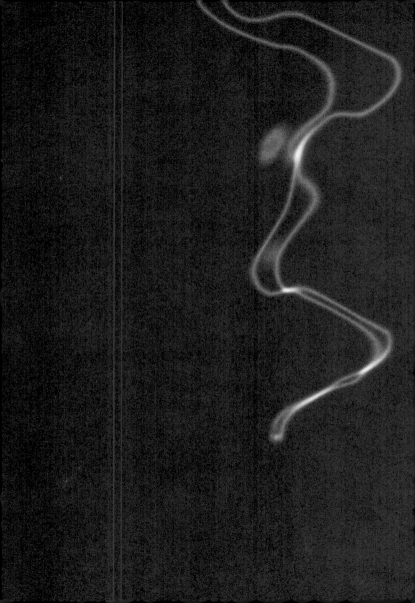

Listen to your HEAD and HEART.
If you decide in an honest, calm, and sane
way that you will not fight for your life,

it is your right.

May you live the remainder of your life
on your own terms, with a minimum
of suffering, among those who
care about you.

We know that the sharing of our lives
is soon to end, but we can continue to be
for each other what we have always been—
as well as what we wanted but
sometimes failed to be.

—   DR. ADRIAAN VERWOERDT   —

Communicating with the Fatally Ill

And, in case these words were not whispered in your ear at birth, or in case they were and somehow you've allowed yourself to forget them along the way— please remember this.

Use your time

wisely...

...and when your time comes to die,
you'll know that your soul
can rest in peace.

Meanwhile,

as you live each day...

You may find that a few things remain to
be finished—*perhaps a number of things*—
that might complete your life.

Before you know it,
you may even discover many new things
that you want from life...

go

Pray to God but row
for shore.

RUSSIAN PROVERB

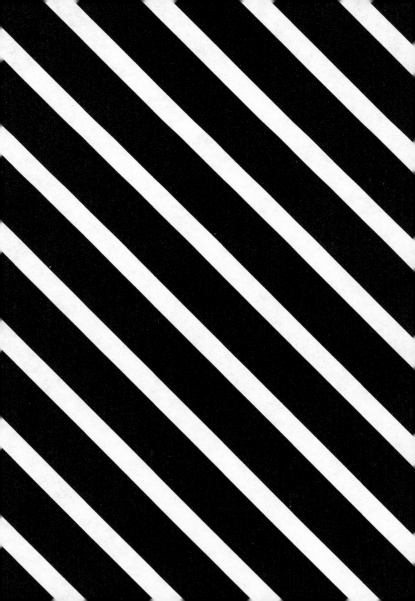

This is an invitation to live the rest of your life

well.

If you're like most of us,

you have probably made plenty of mistakes in your life up to this point. We all have regrets or, at least, recognize that we could have done some things differently.

However, if you can honestly

accept the choices that you've made in your life, then your passing— though sad and disappointing to your survivors—

will be that much easier.

Dying at peace,
WHENEVER it is your time to die,
is a worthwhile goal.

It begins with living at peace.

That's where cancer—or any other
life-threatening experience—
can enrich your life.

Illness can provide both the
OPPORTUNITY and the INCENTIVE
that you may need to get
your life in order.

heal to become sound or healthy again.
Oxford Concise Dictionary

This resolution is called **healing.**
It is a concept you'll hear more about.
Healing has more to do with

love (accepting yourself),

contentment (feeling good about your life),

and **peace** (accepting your mortality)
than it does with any official
pronouncement of physical CURE.

"I am going to die from cancer **but**

I am going to die a healthy man."

V E R N —a cancer patient

This universal need—and search—to find
MEANING and BALANCE in our lives
is more immediately felt with
the specter of death (cancer)
here to simplify your priorities.

Cancer interrupts your daily activities
and forces you to

look

at your life more closely.

There will be no mistaking the

flash of insight...

For a brief moment time stops.
It then resumes, but with somewhat
less certainty because you've had this
glimpse of your own mortality.

The change in your perception will be
quite profound because while you may
expect that your life will now begin to
fade, the OPPOSITE is true.

See for yourself.

Your life will suddenly become more vital
THAN EVER BEFORE, as a result of
an extraordinary new

consciousness.

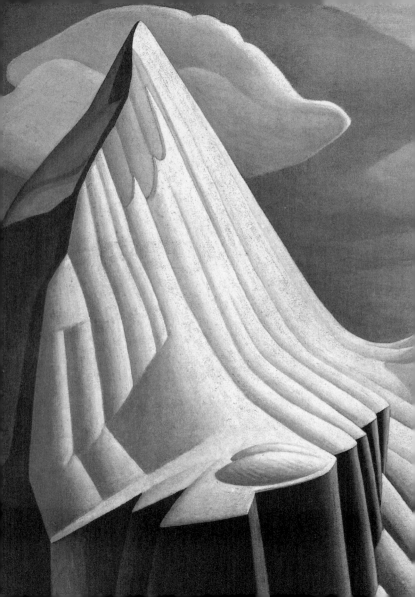

I don't *believe*. I KNOW.

— UNATTRIBUTED —

Lawren S. Harris (1885–1970) *Mount Lefroy* (detail), 1930
Oil on canvas, 133.5 × 153.5 cm
McMichael Canadian Art Collection, Kleinburg, Ontario
With the kind permission of Mrs. Margaret Knox

Despite your newfound appreciation for life, it is NATURAL that you will sometimes think about dying, too.

This tension between living and dying is normal and expected.

"The fundamental tension of opposites, I think, is the **struggle**— especially when you're seriously ill— between wanting to live and wishing to die."

from *Letting Go: Morrie's Reflections on Living While Dying*, by

M O R R I E   S C H W A R T Z

—professor and author who lived with Lou Gehrig's Disease

Workers stop for a lunch break atop a steel girder high above New York City during the construction of the Empire State Building. Completed in 1931—in an astonishing 2 years— it became the world's tallest building at 381 m. (1,250 ft.) and held this record until 1973.
©CORBIS / Bettmann

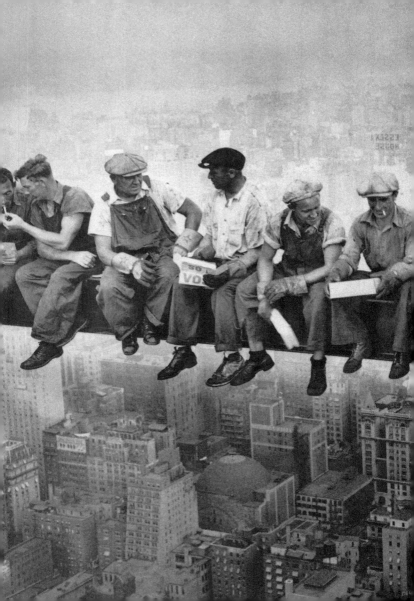

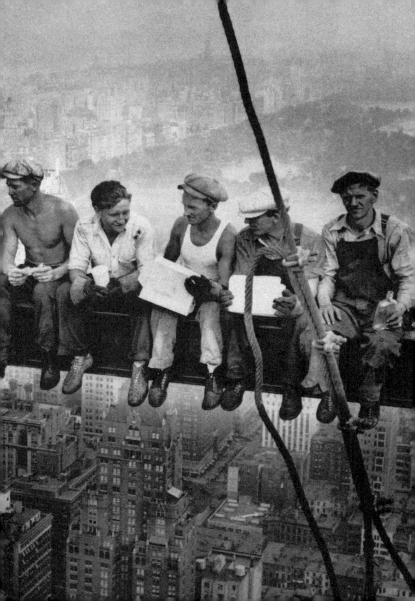

No matter what you might fear,
and the state of your health,
when all is said and done,
the situation is pretty obvious...

"You can EITHER live for the rest of your life,

OR die for the rest of your life."

DR. JOSEPH CONNORS

—systemic oncologist, associate professor, chairman of tumor group

With thoughts about death on your mind, it will take **nerve** to speak about your future life, especially if you look and feel critically ill, and if your prognosis is discouraging.

Don't worry about looking unrealistic. Thinking about your own survival will help to redirect your focus from dying to living.

It COULD ALSO help you to outlive everyone's expectations.

"It is important to picture a future for yourself
that acknowledges the **uncertainty** that exists.
Uncertainty allows hope to occur.
AND HOPE IS ESSENTIAL FOR LIFE."

KATHY BODELL —clinical nurse specialist, palliative care

We don't exist in isolation.

You can be influenced emotionally—
POSITIVELY AND NEGATIVELY—by
those caring for you and visiting.
Sometimes it will be a challenge to
overcome *their* personal fears
regarding *your* health.

Don't give up on me.
Like you, I'm here.
I'm alive.

And right now,

"PLEASE listen to what I am saying! LISTENING TO ME would be the finest thing that you could do in order to help me get through this ordeal."

this IS my life!

The uncertainty in your life can create an emotional roller-coaster for you and for those around you. On top of this, few of us outside the healthcare system have frontline caregiving experience.

What exactly do YOU need
and expect from others?

If you are having a GOOD DAY,
then bright, cheerful encouragement
might be best for you.

Conversely, on a BAD DAY,
this same cheerful response from others
might feel trite or condescending—you
may be desperate for acknowledgment
of just how serious things are.

I don't choose to be walking.

I don't choose to be talking.

The only thing I'm choosing

is to lie here woozy-snoozing

So won't you kindly go away.

I am NOT going to get up today!

— DR. SEUSS —

I Am Not Going to Get Up Today!

You deserve kindness, compassion, care,
dignity, times of despair, times of denial,
and the FREEDOM to live life—
on your own terms—in your own way.

You also deserve your birthright—
access to the enormous well of personal
POWER that is within you. We all
have it. *Some of us need to reclaim it.*

If you want to get well, the major
contributing factor will be the

POWER OF YOUR WILL.

believe accept as true or
conveying truth.
Oxford Concise Dictionary

For the best results: Strive to be
optimistic in your outlook, and project
your health *whenever* you can.

YOU MUST BELIEVE that your chosen
therapy is going to help you, and that you
have a chance to get well, otherwise you'll
be using your energy to fight
your treatment, instead of your cancer.

Sometimes you'll be DEVASTATED.
Despite the sometimes grim reality, try to
switch back to some personal TRIGGER—
an image, thought, prayer, loved one, or
whatever—that gives you **strength.**

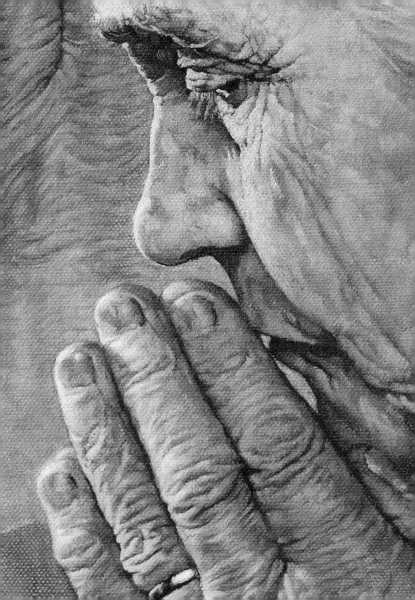

Hope is a journey, not a destination;

its value lies in the exploration.

Hope is the way we live life and the

journey of hope should last until we end.

— DAVID KESSLER —

The Rights of the Dying

The good news is that
there's always **hope** that you will
feel well again—lots of people
with cancer do.

If you look, you will find

living

proof.

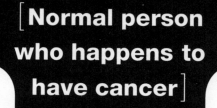

Here are some ideas
for cancer

SURVIVORS

in training.

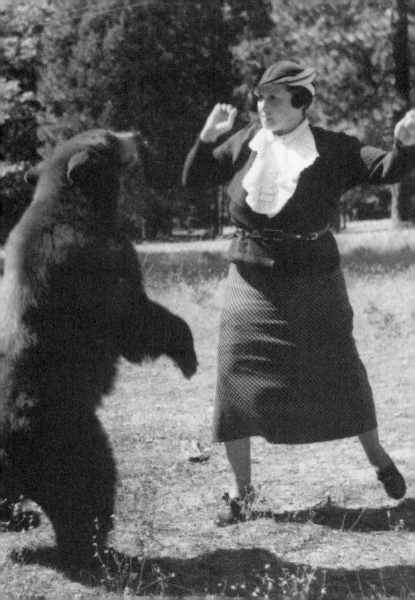

1

Expect to keep on living.

Long live oncologists and their patients.

2

Find well-qualified healthcare professionals that you like *and can trust* to help you.

And give them your own trust, effort, and respect.

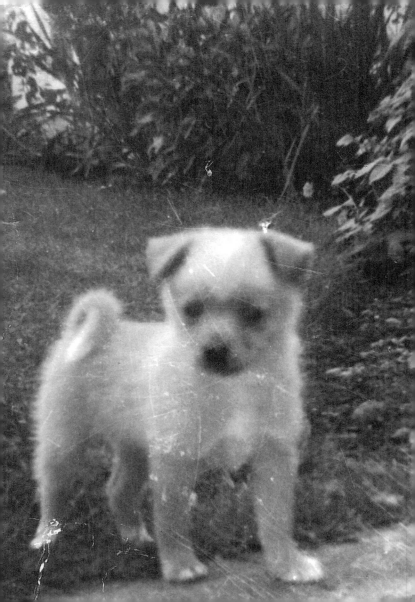

3

Create

an environment

for WELLNESS.

Surround yourself only with
WHOEVER AND WHATEVER
you feel will contribute to your rest,
strength, and inspiration.

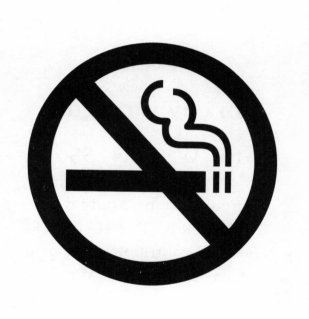

4

STOP doing things that

may have contributed

to your disease

or may be jeopardizing your
present health.

A fool is a person
who keeps on doing the same thing
and expects different results.

— ALBERT EINSTEIN —

[E A T   Y O U R 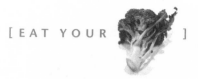]

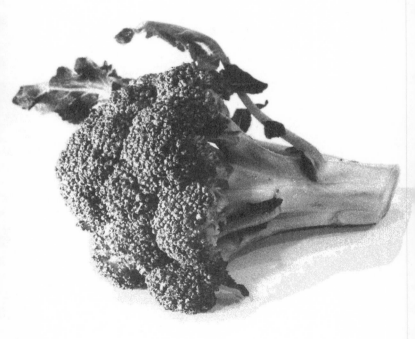

Broccoli is a great source of fiber, calcium, potassium, and a compound called sulphoraphane that has been identified with cancer prevention.

5

START doing things that will *contribute to* your health.

Engage in practices that respect your BODY and your MIND.

Alison Edwards & Kent Bodell   *The Broccoli Follies,* 1999
Black and white photographs
©Alison Edwards & Kent Bodell

I NEED help!

6

Make GOOD

communication

a priority.

Learn to communicate your
feelings honestly, respectfully,
and effectively.

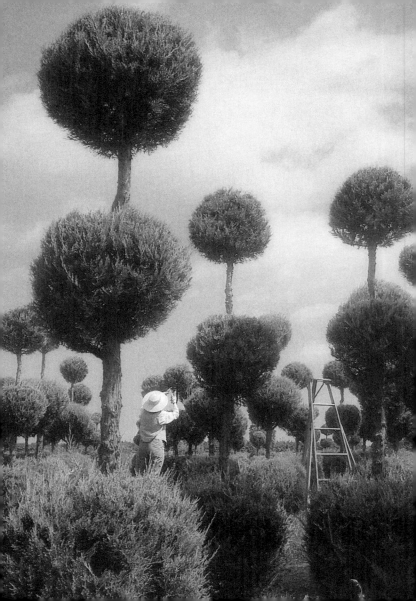

mantra a word or sound repeated
to aid concentration in meditation,
orig. in Hinduism.
Oxford Concise Dictionary

7

Find TOOLS that will help you achieve your health objectives.

Explore visualization and relaxation
techniques, dream journals,
retreats, affirmations, mantras,
meditation, music, art therapy—or
whatever seems right for YOU.

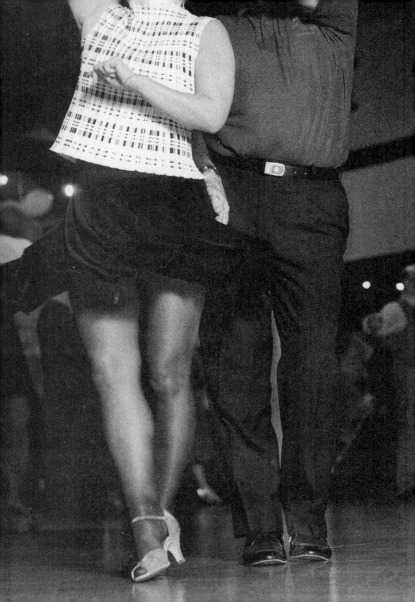

8

MOVE your body as much as you *possibly* can.

Physical activity helps promote the production of endorphins in the brain— those natural stimulants that help boost your energy level and your spirits.

Medical fact tells us that EVEN HEALTHY PEOPLE, when confined to bed for a week, will lose a great deal of physical strength *and bone mass.*

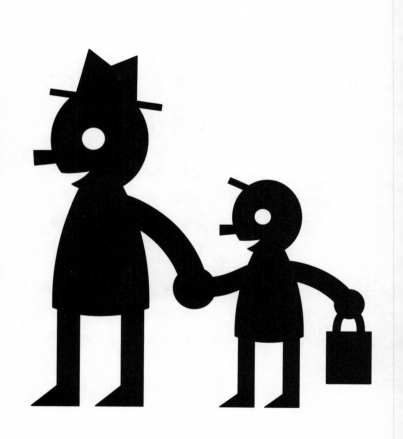

9

NURTURE the quality

of your life.

If of thy mortal goods thou art bereft,

And from thy slender store

two loaves alone to thee are left,

Sell one, and with the dole

Buy hyacinths to feed thy soul.

— SHAIKH MUSLIH-UD-DIN SA'DI —

From Gulistan: The Rose Garden

Mike Lee *Man and Child,* 1993
Digital illustration
©Mike Lee

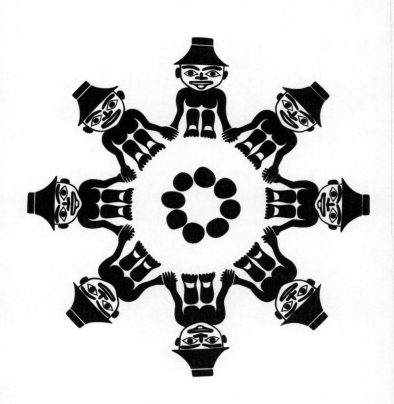

10

Seek the spiritual resources that suit you.

You do not have to go through this alone.
Let your intuition guide you to the
kind of support that YOU need
to get through this.

It is often necessary to make a decision on

the basis of knowledge sufficient for action

but insufficient to satisfy the intellect.

— IMMANUEL KANT —

Beau Dick (Kwakwaka'wakw) *Sacred Circle,* 1992
Painting originally created for a ceremonial drum honoring the return of the once out-
lawed traditional Potlatch. A gift to his daughter, Kerri Lynne, the image depicts rekindling
the fire of Haida spirit, culture, and purpose in a new generation of young Haida People.
©Beau Dick / With the kind permission of Kerri Lynne Dick

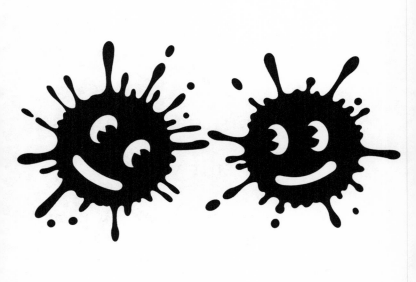

11

Laugh for health.

I never forget a face,

but in your case

I'll be glad to make an exception.

— GROUCHO MARX —

The Splat Brothers, c. 1986
Ink on film
©From the Studio of Vigon Seireeni

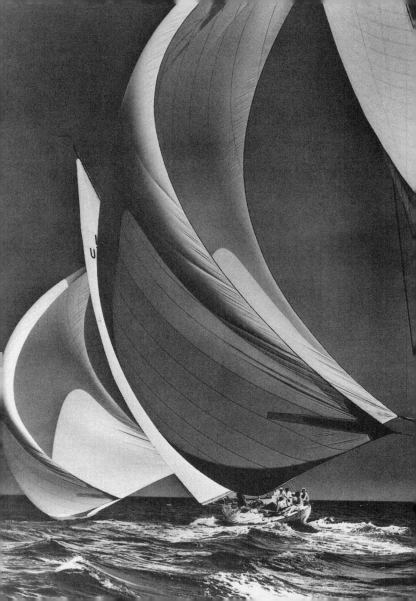

12

Stay focused

but remain flexible.

No wind favors an unknown port.

— PROVERB —

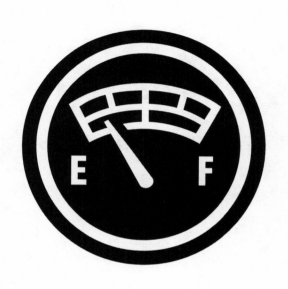

13

Pace yourself *realistically.*

You'll LEARN to be responsive to your changing mental, emotional, and physical energy levels.

RIGHT NOW, it is easy to "overdo it." When you do, your body will let you know it—BIGTIME.

For every action there is an equal and opposite reaction.

— NEWTON'S THIRD LAW OF MOTION —

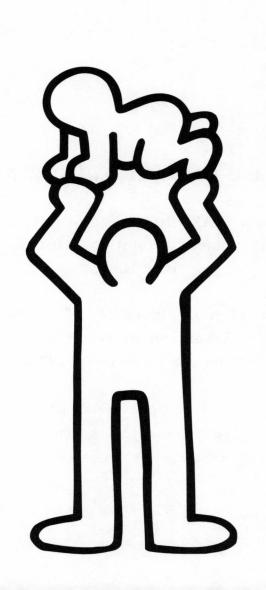

14

Stay connected to PEOPLE and they will give you strength.

It is a well-known fact that people who have close personal relationships tend to *live longer* than those who feel that they are alone in the world.

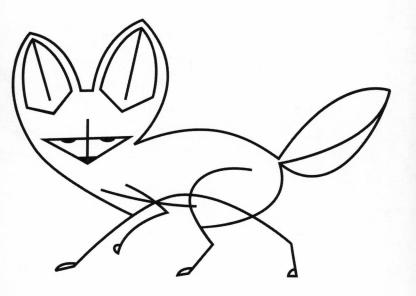

15

Listen carefully to the advice offered to you but ALWAYS use your own discretion.

"Is this the procedure that you would recommend for YOUR OWN MOTHER?"

JACQUELINE OSBORNE —longtime cancer survivor and teacher

Carlos Aponte *Untitled*
Digital illustration
©Carlos Aponte / EyeWire

You'll want to consider what exactly,
if anything, *you are prepared to do*
in order to help yourself get well again.

Reading and research will tell you
what factors can CONTRIBUTE
to your recovery. You'll also learn that
there are several factors which can
INTERFERE with your recovery.

While lack of social support,
love, money, and time can challenge you,
much can be achieved through your own
courage, patience, hope,
and self-discipline.

Overcoming cancer is an important personal challenge and will require your FULL COMMITMENT.

If you're serious about getting well, there are any number of **tools** you can use to help you but this one is *invaluable*.

It will give you an immediate energy boost...

Go ahead, list some of the reasons
why you want to live.

(Any order will do.)

_____

_____

_____

_____

_____

_____

Need more space to write?

_____

_____

_____

_____

_____

_____

Now choose from these

THE MAIN REASON

why you want to live.

*It should fill you with inspiration
and with hope.*

(It may be quite general or very specific.)

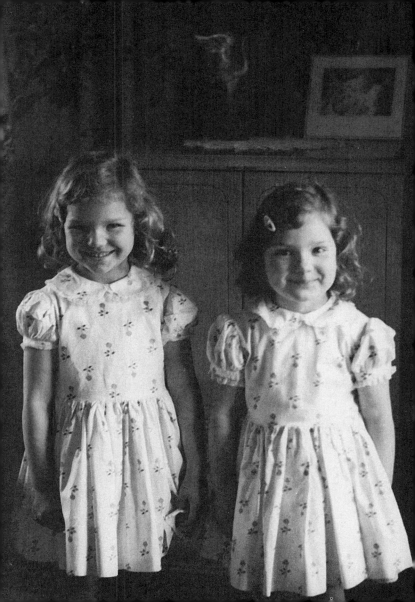

It is much easier to live if someone
loves or needs you, or you love or need
someone or something. A cat,
a dog, a spouse, a friend, a child,
a caregiver will do.

If this reason is intensely personal,
you may wish to keep it tucked in your
journal or commit it to memory.

If you're not so shy, maybe you'd rather
tape a copy of it to a prominent wall, or
ask a friend to mount a huge sign outside
your window, where you, and your
neighbors, can see it clearly

every single day!

If you feel that you have no one, be sure to make an extra effort to care for yourself until others present themselves. PEOPLE WILL FIND YOU, IF YOU ALLOW THEM TO.

Be sure that your REASON TO LIVE incorporates the thing(s) in the world that you feel most passionately about.

If you choose carefully,

your GOAL will sustain you.

My Most Important Reason for Living:

_____

We all know that REALITY BEGINS WITH THOUGHT. People who make goals have an opportunity to reach them.

Maybe the reason that you want to live is quite general—for example: you simply value your life. *Or, perhaps...*

Your reason for living includes a specific time element, like the education or wedding of a child, a birthday, or a family reunion.

The element of **time** raises a few issues because time can be flexible.

Time

can seemingly shrink or expand depending upon what you elect to do with it. If something is very important to you, you will more likely find time for it.

There are countless cases of people who—despite the extent of disease within their body—*have lived far beyond what seemed physically possible* in order to fulfill a meaningful goal.

And have then...died.

Living your life fully and with satisfaction
is a MAJOR accomplishment.

One that has brought sublime
peace and contentment
to many individuals and their families.

Some individuals live each day
completely at peace with themselves.

Most of us hope to experience this
UNDERSTANDING before we die.
This endeavor becomes our life's journey.

COMPLETION

of your own GOALS, however modest,
may mark the end of your visualization,
and signal that your *life* is complete.

You may experience a tremendous
sense of relief once you resolve
what you feel was unfinished business.

You may further sense that
THE TIME IS NOW RIGHT FOR YOU
to let go of life.

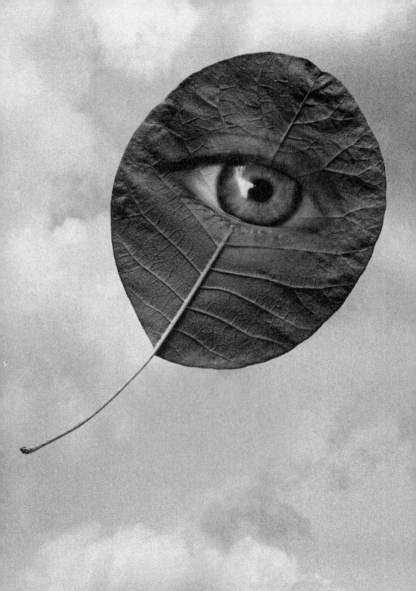

That afternoon, in the golden light of dusk,

Daniel let go. He fell effortlessly.

He seemed to smile peacefully, as he fell.

"Goodbye for now, Freddie," he said.

— LEO F. BUSCAGLIA, PH.D. —

The Fall of Freddie the Leaf

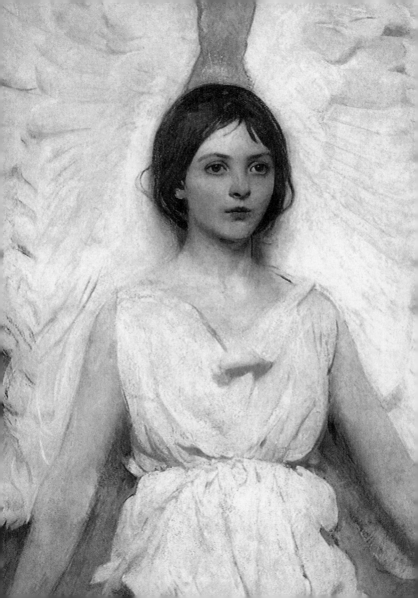

Cancer may encourage
your own *spiritual healing.*

Yet "GETTING WELL"
may mean that while you
will in fact heal,
you may not be CURED
of your disease.

It could be that your body
has PASSED the stage where major
organs are able to regenerate and your
basic systems are failing.

If the disease has spread throughout
your body, you may not have the strength
to do anything for yourself but make your
peace and prepare to die.

Then again—perhaps

this is NOT what you

have in mind for your life.

Sometimes it appears that nothing short of an **unexplainable recovery** can or will stave off the inevitable course of deterioration within your body.

Sometimes this happens.

Go to the library or on the Internet, read about spontaneous remission, remarkable recoveries, and MIRACLES. Talk to doctors who have seen unexplainable RESULTS and visit those people who were once "HOPELESS CASES." Learn about their attitudes, their choices, and their treatments.

Seek encourage

Ask people for

ment and support.

ideas and help.

I'm here with you.
It's going to be all right.
I'm going to help.
How do you feel?

re:so

Do you NEED anything?
What do you WANT to happen?
What can I do?
We'll all pull together.
Is it all right to talk now?
Are you afraid?
Everybody is thinking of you.
They all send their love.
You're really important to me/us.
I KNOW you can do this.

urces

Find someone who

did the "impossible."

Rediscover nature, surround yourself
with music, art, pets, people,
and objects you love.

Seek out mentors and coaches, support

groups and heroes. Find people
who will provide inspiration, and those
who are willing to help you to

fight for your health.

There are many
different personalities, many interests,
and many approaches to cancer
and cancer therapy.

Some are MORE conservative.

Some are LESS conservative.

Ask around, you might be surprised to learn of some of the remarkable things that people with cancer are doing with themselves in order to feel *good*.

While "feeling good" is a process that takes some imagination and some ongoing effort, the results will speak for themselves. Amazing things *can and do happen* when healthcare professionals work closely with patients who are motivated to fight for their health, and who are willing to make the effort to do what's required.

Many of the women did not even know what a dragon boat was before they got involved. These were not elite athletes— they were game middle-aged women who embarked on a rigorous training program.

Abreast In A Boat was the world's first dragon boat team consisting entirely of women living with breast cancer. Formed in 1996 as a research project under the direction of Dr. Don McKenzie at THE UNIVERSITY OF BRITISH COLUMBIA, it boasted 24 cancer patients, ages 33–63.

Despite their high risk for problems, due to removal of underarm lymph nodes, the research team and paddlers bravely (and successfully) challenged conventional wisdom that repetitive strenuous upper body exercise would cause lymphedema— irreversible swelling of the chest or arms.

Video screen capture courtesy Global Television (Vancouver), from the 1998 documentary *Through Fire and Water: The Story of Abreast In A Boat*.
With permission of the Abreast In A Boat Society

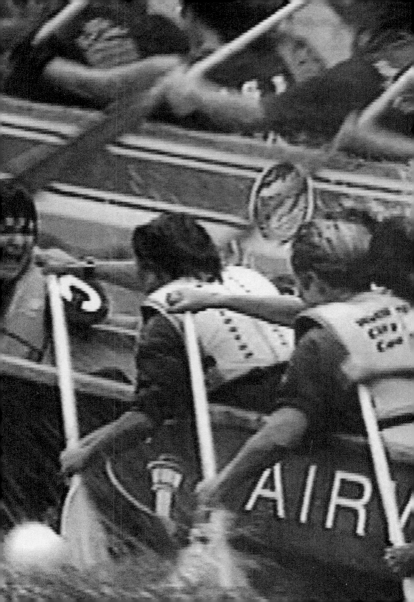

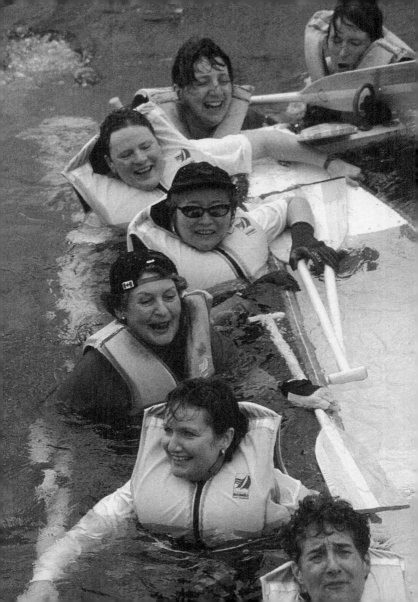

DRAGON BOAT RACING derives from an ancient Chinese ceremony that symbolizes man's struggle with nature, and his fight against deadly enemies.

"On their first international dragon boat meet in Wellington Harbour, New Zealand, the women of Abreast In A Boat were terrified. Despite their coaches' wisdom and the athletes' best efforts, the wind [won] the first round as a stiff gust [toppled] the racers into the water during their first two practice runs."

Undaunted by the rough seas that dumped them, the women braved their races against far more experienced international dragon boat teams. In the end, their courage won hearts, earned respect, and inspired people facing challenges worldwide.

Excerpts above courtesy of Global Television (Vancouver) as quoted in the 1998 documentary *Through Fire and Water: The Story of Abreast In A Boat.*
Photograph : Vern Blair *Sheila, Kate, Diane, Esther, Carol, Donna & Anne, 1997*
Members of the Abreast In A Boat Team, capsized in Wellington Harbour, await their tow.
©Vern Blair / The Abreast In A Boat Society

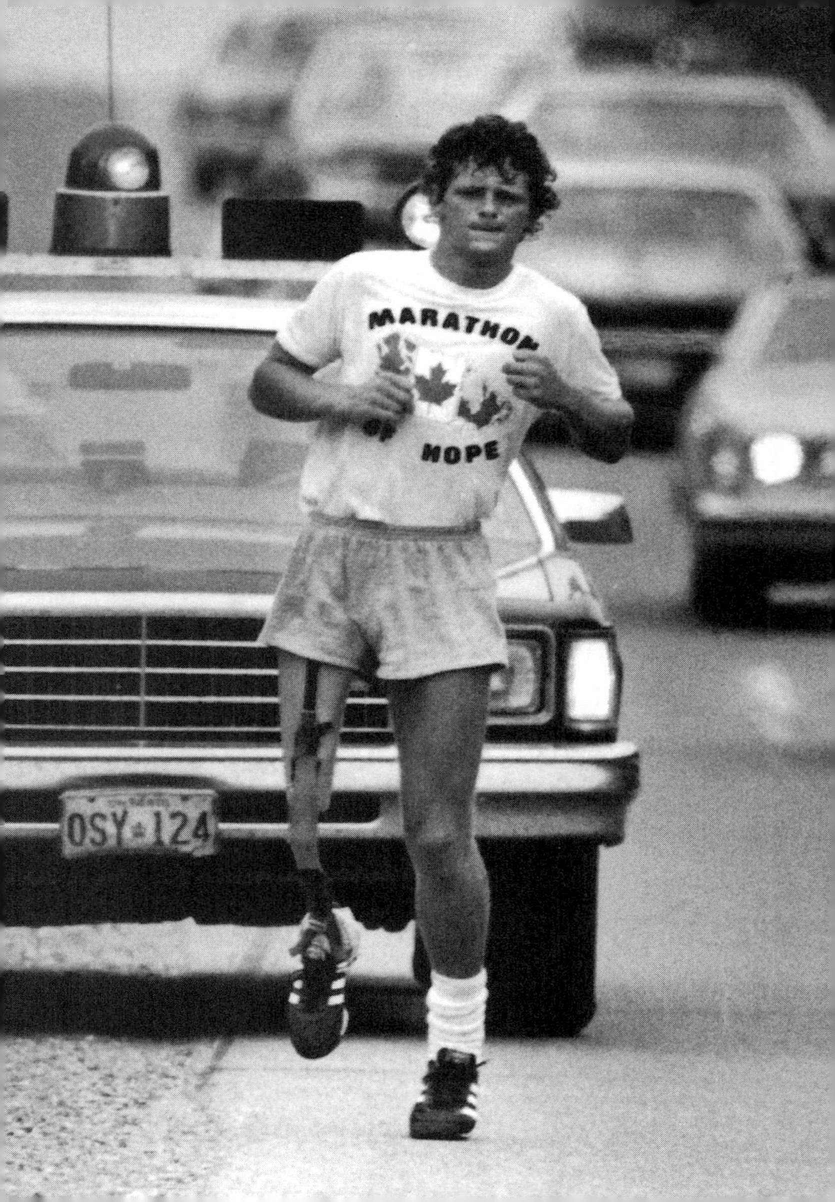
MARATHON
HOPE
OSY 124

The Marathon of Hope

was the dream of an 18-year-old university
student from British Columbia
named Terry Fox.

Terry wanted to run 5,300 miles across
Canada—from sea to sea—in order to
raise $1 toward cancer research for each
Canadian. His spirit inspired a nation.

In 1980, less than two years after losing
his right leg 6 inches above the knee
to a rare bone cancer (osteogenic sarcoma),
Terry was running at least a marathon
a day (26 miles) on a prosthetic limb.

Gail Harvey *Terry Fox, The Marathon of Hope* (detail), 1980
Black and white photograph
©1999 Gail Harvey / The Terry Fox Foundation

He quickly became a beloved international hero. After months of remarkable courage and physical pain, having conquered almost two-thirds of the challenge (3,339 miles), Terry was forced to stop the run. The cancer had metastasized to both lungs.

Cancer took his life, but not before Terry and his courageous Marathon of Hope had raised over $20 million.

The Terry Fox Foundation continues his legacy for cancer research in over 50 countries through the commitment of hundreds of thousands of supporters worldwide.

Diagnosed in 1996 with testicular
cancer that metastasized to his
stomach, lungs, and brain, this
27-year-old elite cyclist underwent
surgery, radiation, and chemotherapy
and waged a courageous fight for his
health.

I had the same emotions when I was sick as I have
as a competitive athlete. At first I was angry; [then] I
felt motivated and driven get better. And then when
I knew I was getting better, I knew I was winning.

LANCE ARMSTRONG — cyclist, cancer survivor,

winner of the 1999 Tour de France, founder of the Lance Armstrong Foundation

On July 25, 1999, American cyclist
Lance Armstrong won the Tour de
France in Paris. He dominated the gruelling
21-day tour, winning four race stages
outright—only the 4th rider to do so in the
event's 86-year history. A stunning achieve-
ment made even more remarkable because
Lance is a cancer survivor. His triumphant
international return *ignited* the world.

Perhaps these stories are too **BIG**, and too intimidating to inspire you.

Remember this:
There are many, many ORDINARY PEOPLE with cancer who do small and extraordinary things every day.

And there are those who help them.

Those who are here, give their sharing.
Small amounts or great, it is sufficient.

— GERALDINE MARIE PAPAN —

God's Winter

The best thing that

YOU can do

to take control of what is happening
is to CHALLENGE YOUR CANCER by
harnessing your inner resources—

the strength of your **Mind,** and

the strength of your **Body.**

Some people, elite athletes for example, *already work with the connection between*

the mind and the body.

You won't surprise them with biofeedback techniques any more than you would patients who have learned to control their blood pressure, migraines, or heart rate, or those who have firewalked.

And you're certainly not going to tell recovered "hopeless cases" anything THEY don't already know.

A short course in mind-body discipline may be enormously helpful to your healing, and to pain/stress management.

However, MASTERING mind-body techniques is usually the result of much commitment, self-discipline, and practice. It is probably unrealistic to expect any significant progress in this area without adequate training.

Despite sincere intentions, *your efforts may do little* to arrest the actual progression of disease within your body.

One of the frightening things about cancer, it brings with it a looming deadline, yet great *uncertainty*.

PROGNOSIS

"So, really...

STATISTICS

how much

SURVIVAL RATE

time

SURVIVAL TIME

DO

REMISSION

I

RECURRENCE

have?"

Don't expect anyone to know
how long you will live.

"I don't need to speak for God. God can speak for Himself."

REVEREND COLIN JOHNSTONE —cancer center chaplain

Oncologists are often asked this difficult
question and are reluctant to give you
an answer (based on their experience)
because NO ONE CAN PREDICT YOUR
DEATH WITH CERTAINTY.

If you've bullied your physician for
a GUESS, take it as such.

Who knows?!

Cancer isn't the only way to end a life,
and it certainly doesn't give you—
or anyone else—IMMUNITY.

A person with cancer could be killed
any number of ways, on any given day,
just like anyone else.

God is dead. —*Nietzsche*   **Nietzsche is dead.** —*God*

— ANONYMOUS GRAFFITI WRITER —

Off the Wall: Graffiti for the Soul

Be smart.

Look both ways before you
cross the street.

In other words,

take care of yourself.

CITY GREENERY

If you should happen after dark

to find yourself in Central Park,

Ignore the paths that beckon you

And hurry, hurry to the zoo,

And creep into the tiger's lair.

Frankly, you'll be safer there.

— OGDEN NASH —

Our City, Our Citizens from *Everyone but Me and Thee*

Birth and death

define our lives.

Show respect for your life but accept that death, like birth, is natural. It is an inevitable part of the cycle for human beings, NOT some sad, terrible failure.

PREPAREDNESS is what we mean when we say that possible or imminent death may give you a new way to

look at your life.

Does it matter?
Does *anything* matter?
Or...
Does *everything* matter?

What is the measure of
"a good life"?

This is the age-old question.

We all have a different journey.

But at the end of life, if you can
claim peace within yourself,
without being consumed by doubts,
regrets, and loneliness, you'll find that

YOUR LIFE has **meaning.**

*That's what all this talk of healing is
about—experiencing acceptance, peace, love,
joy, and compassion.*

That's it.

Even if you feel that you
never did much with your life,
it is MORE THAN ENOUGH
if those around you
have benefited
from having known you,
from having been
touched by you.

Whether it is cancer that kills you,
or some other disease, an accident,
or old age, matters little.

The *real gift* of experiencing

life-threatening illness

is that you have

the *opportunity* to confront

your own mortality in time...

...to feel all right

about your life
and if necessary, in time to heal
what it is that ails you—in your soul
as well as your body—

before you die.

As for you Rebel Cells,

I've only recently come to appreciate

what you've done for me.

Painful as it was, you made me THINK!

— JÜRGEN GROHNE —

Talking to Your Cells: The Cancer Microperspective

You've been given a good chance to

understand the Meaning of Life

while you're still alive!

The best thing that could happen
to you is that you use this time to get

completely current in your life.

You resolve all your relationships
and make peace with yourself, as well
as the rest of the world.

love an intense feeling of deep affection or fondness for a person or thing.
Oxford Concise Dictionary

If you haven't already, you could experience love.

Non Nobis Solum Not for Ourselves Alone

— THE SISTERS OF ST. ANN —

Motto: St. Joseph's School of Nursing

Kathy Boake W. *Posey,* 1999
Ruby cut, 10.16 cm × 12.70 cm
©K. Boake W.

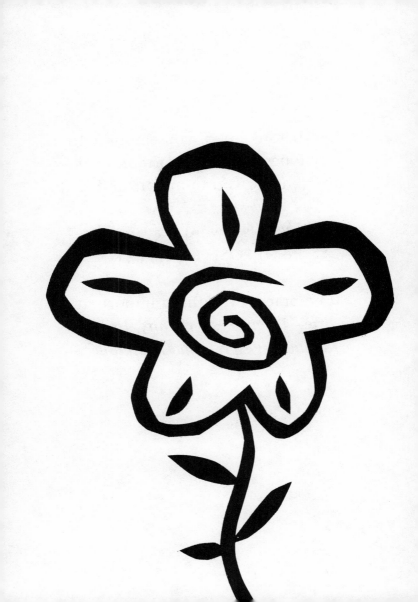

Now, before any of you emotionally shy types get uncomfortable, it is important for you to understand that

love is a word that means the OPPOSITE OF FEAR.

It embraces everything important in life—*Forgiveness, Dignity, Honesty, Kindness, Respect, and Acceptance.*

I hope when your time comes to die,
YOUR HEART will be filled
with gratitude and love for life.

To die healed, not wounded;

peaceful, not angry;

grateful, not resentful;

with love, not fear...

These are major achievements.

And what if you live

for a long time, yet?

What doesn't kill you makes you stronger.

— ALBERT CAMUS —

Probably **much** stronger.
And probably much happier, too.

If you want a jump start to get your
life in order, here is an exercise that is a

guaranteed fast track

to peace of mind *in your lifetime.*

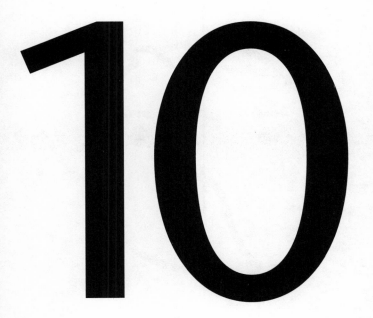

10

STEPS TO PEACE OF MIND

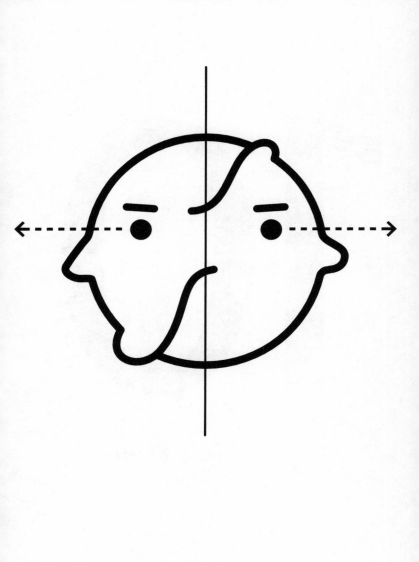

Janus *is the Greek God*
with two faces—one young and one old.
The wise old man looks back upon
past experiences while the young man,
filled with the optimism of youth,
looks expectantly toward the future.

You, too, can benefit from such vision
and enjoy guaranteed PEACE OF MIND
by completing the deceptively simple
exercise that follows.

Miriam MacPhail & abcotter@home *The Contemplation of Janus,* 1996
Digital illustration
©Miriam MacPhail and Arlene Cotter

In one hour or less,

use the following pages to
write down your IMMEDIATE ideas
about what things would help to
make your life complete.

*These goals should be both personal
and achievable.*

Keep the process intuitive.

Avoid rationalization and censorship.

*Don't make the exercise any more
complex than it needs to be.*

This exercise is DEFINITELY WORTH THE EFFORT. (If it seems intimidating or too physically demanding for you, you may want to ask a friend for help.)

Apologize to someone...

Get help to write a long-overdue letter...

Swim in the ocean...

Play the piano and sing with friends...

Surrender a family secret...

Ask someone for help...

Look at your old photographs...

Call the end to a feud...

Formalize your will...

Arrange a holiday...

Give away some of your possessions...

Tell someone that you love them...

Go fishing...

Contact old friends and relatives...

Make a videotape for your loved ones...

Write **10** items
(important doesn't mean big)
in random order, as the thoughts
occur to you.

Remove just ONE item
(the most expendable) each time
that you rewrite the list.

Forget about neatness here—
go for accuracy—cross-outs and
scribbles are natural.

TEN THINGS TO DO BEFORE I DIE

1

2

3

4

5

6

7

8

9

10

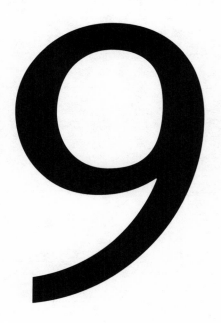

NINE THINGS TO DO BEFORE I DIE

1
2
3
4
5
6
7
8
9

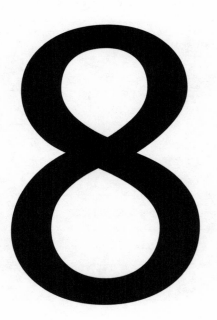

EIGHT THINGS TO DO BEFORE I DIE

1

2

3

4

5

6

7

8

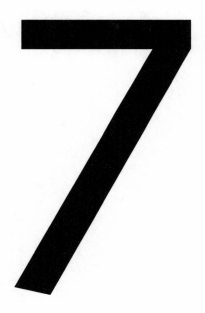

SEVEN THINGS TO DO BEFORE I DIE

1

2

3

4

5

6

7

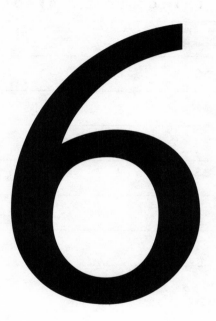

SIX THINGS TO DO BEFORE I DIE

1

2

3

4

5

6

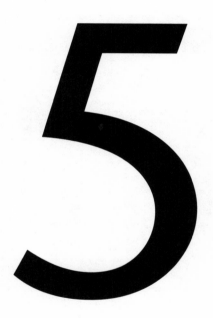

FIVE THINGS TO DO BEFORE I DIE

1

2

3

4

5

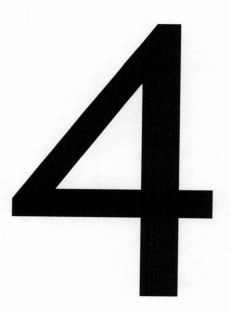

FOUR THINGS TO DO BEFORE I DIE

1

2

3

4

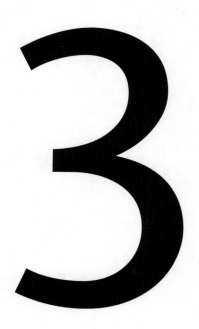

THREE THINGS TO DO BEFORE I DIE

1 _____

2 _____

3 _____

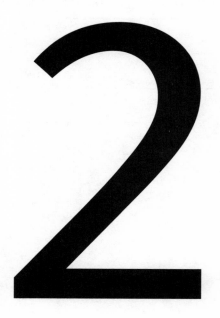

TWO THINGS TO DO BEFORE I DIE

1 _____

2 _____

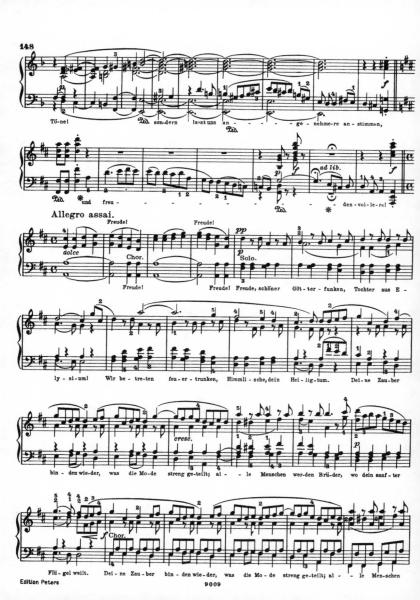

THE **MOST** IMPORTANT THING

TO DO BEFORE I DIE

1

↑

START HERE

The Ninth Symphony in D Minor, Opus 125, An die Freude (Ode to Joy)
Based on Friedrich Schiller's *Ode – Choral Symphony,* Fourth Movement: 66 minutes
Composed by Ludwig van Beethoven (1770 – 1827)
Symphonien Für Klavier (Zu Handen)
Reprinted by permission of C. F. Peters Corporation, New York

If you're reading this then you have all the time you need to feel well because the power REALLY lies in STATING AND RELEASING YOUR HEART'S DESIRE.

People who are diagnosed with cancer often describe their ordeal as
a profound gift—
one that forced them to focus on what is essential in life.

What you have just created is a list of things that you feel will help you to heal what it is that ails you.

Address the items on your list in order of priority, and you'll add QUALITY to your life.

Guaranteed.

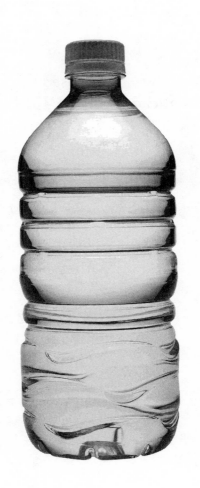

Go ahead, drink of Life.

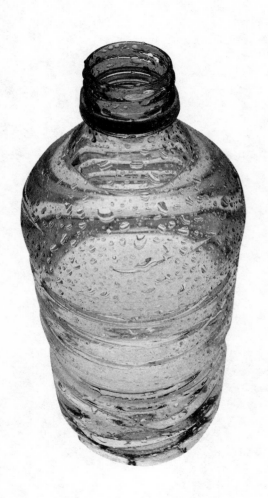

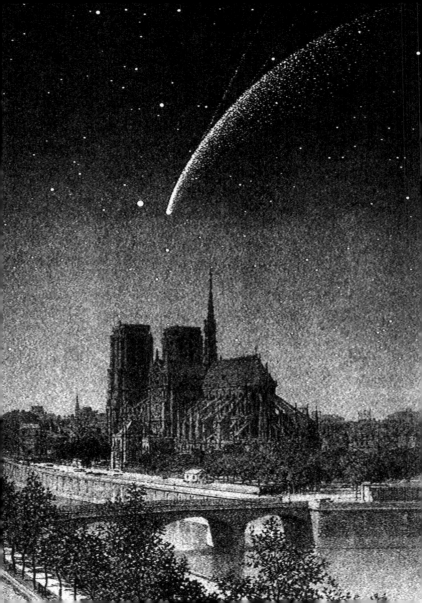

Even **if** the doctor does not give you a year,

even if he hesitates about a month,

make one brave push

and see what can be accomplished

in a week.

— ROBERT LOUIS STEVENSON —

Virginibus Puerisque

Donati Comet Over Notre Dame by Amedée Guillemin, c. 1858

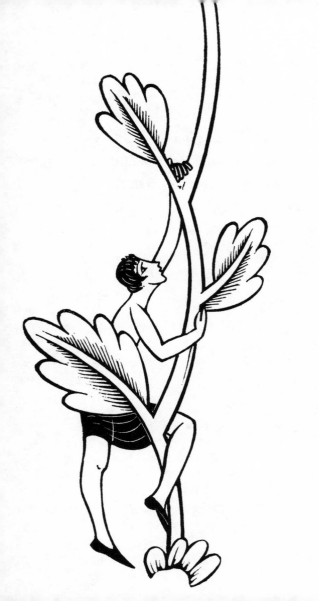

This is the **end** of the book but

the **beginning** of

the rest of your life.

Eric Gill (1882 – 1940) *Boy About to Climb Tree* (detail), 1929 – 31
Wood engraving, 19.9 × 5.6 cm Decorative border for *The Canterbury Tales*
The Art Collection, The Harry Ransom Humanities Research Center,
The University of Texas at Austin
With kind permission of the Eric Gill Estate

I didn't get well alone and I didn't write this book alone. *From This Moment On* represents what I have learned with the help of others. It reflects the collective wisdom, skill, inspiration, and love of many individuals who at some time said or did the right thing—people who offered their time, talent, prayers, energy, and hope to help me get through my own cancer diagnosis and make this book a reality. I don't know how they knew what to do—*but they did*.

What follows is only a partial list of
the wise and generous individuals who have
helped me on my own healing journey.

To my indomitable agent Denise Bukowski who made this happen. To my editor at Random House, NY Courtney Hodell who understands the big picture and still minds the small one, and who I thank for giving me everything I needed to make this book. To four individuals who have the ability to look at something in a raw state and see potential— Jürgen Grohne, Maurice Egan, Elma Heidemann, and Randi Gunther. I am grateful to each of them for their kind interest and their invaluable contribution to early drafts. To Don Atkins who forced many people to read the manuscript on my behalf and who I just like—a lot. To Victor Marks for his early encouragement and generous advice. It gave me the confidence that I needed to continue. To Steve Cobb who always takes the time to roll up his sleeves and help. To Barbara Hodgson who offered early critical feedback and answered all my questions with infinite patience. To Dr. Michael Harlos whose careful and detailed review of the early manuscript shaped a much kinder book. To my oncologist Dr. Joseph Connors who told me that he was going to do everything in his power to help me overcome my cancer—and who did precisely that. To Jan Gledstone who further cheers my heart. To the fine nurses at the BC Cancer Agency in Vancouver—especially my "first ones": Libby Hager and Iris Isla. To "Marguerite" a sweet nurse at Vancouver Health and Sciences Hospital. To my dear and patient father Julius Cotter who first asked me whether or not I wanted to live and has since then gently guided me back toward life...again and again. To my dear mother Izolda Kovacs Cotter whose faith and love for me have never once wavered. To my sister Linda Holmes who would give her life for my own. Linda willed this book into existence and never gave up her mission to keep me alive. To my big sister Kathy Bodell whose phenomenal 11th-hour contribution made this a much stronger book. She kept me afloat at the end. To Joyce Guy who graciously cared for the difficult recluse in her home, and to her family, especially Elaine Burke and Gwynne MacIntosh. To Dr. Pippa Hawley who offered the most humane introduction to cancer that any patient could ask for and also to Dr. Wakefield. To Sarah Sample who was there in the shadows. To Joseph Biro and his wife Irene who (after some 25 years) made a special trip as soon as they heard that I had cancer. Joe spent less than an hour telling me everything that I needed to know about what was going to happen next. I can't be certain that he didn't say all the things in the book during that short course on living. To the quiet and extraordinary Grand Master Peng who offered healing thanks to Ann Gardner-Vigh and Béla Vigh. To Jürgen Grohne my parallel, mentor, and muse, and a man after my own heart. What I write and think is only better for his tireless involvement and endless ideas. To Frank Sartori the dear man who literally saved my life by refusing to let me die. He is my angel on this earth. To Grace Sartori who offered me her hand when I stumbled. To the Aballini Family, especially Ida, Frank, and Susan who taught me about kindness and spinach-ricotta gnocchi. To my dear friend Miriam MacPhail who deftly edited early drafts and whose intelligence and contribution I am truly grateful for. To my friends Maggie and John Edwards-Pinel who offered the benefit of their considerable publishing experience for both the proposal and the manuscript. To Margaret Braun & Dr. Steve Jordan and the entire Braun Family who encouraged this book (and me) in every way possible. To dear friend Josie Patterson and Norma Lee. To Nanci and Roy Walkup and the rest of the Group for their constant support of my sister Linda, and also of me. To Dr. Joan Chlebowski who gave helpful early feedback and Dr. Rowan Chlebowski who challenged me to maintain momentum until the final page. To Nola George who has a heart as big as the sea and who prayed endlessly for me. To Michele Finnegan who patiently and compassionately found a way to help me re-enter the world. I am deeply grateful. To Lisa Marginson who spotted an opening and guided me toward it. To Dr. Arianna Yakirov-Jarvis who opened the door inch by inch, and finally helped me to slip through it. To Ian Bailey & Erin Hanrahan who showed infinite grace when, without a moment's hesitation, they put my health before any mortgage concerns. To Gary & Mary Hiscox who would not let me become invisible and who generously shared their friends, including the lovely and smart Mary O'Donovan. To some of the friends and colleagues who helped tie me to the world by a thin thread—Kathleen Speakman & Leslie Uyeda, Cilla Bachop, George Vaitkunas, Linda Bartz, Deborah Shackleton, David Hornblow, Roberto Docil, Diana Becker, Kim Blanchette, Gary Miles, Patricia McSherry, Miles Walker, Betsy Jones and Gus Tsetsekes, who I thank for coaxing me to design again. To Patrick Lyndon who knew all about this book and encouraged me to sing about new rooms and blue rooms. To Katharina Duerst and Raef Grohne who have consistently been my friends. To Rolf and Monika Grohne whose enthusiasm for life is simply infectious. To Pat Grohne for her encouragement and review. To Frithjoff Grohne for going to bat for me one fine day. To Effie Klein, a producer at Global TV, for her great contribution. To Kim Schachte

& Lloyd Bernhardt for the long and generous computer loan when I had no equipment nor resources. To Chris & Karin Hall who dared to visit when I said "no visitors!" and later let me stay at their pretty home. To the Pollak Family, the Sutherland Family, the Papan Family and the Czotter Family who remembered me. To Dr. Tim Yeomans a physician and a healer, who listens very carefully and continues to guide me through my own healing journey. To Debra Allman who gives further nudges. To the many individuals who allowed me to include their words, quotations, and art—especially Brian Cronin whose early permission paved the way for much talent to come. To Mrs. Margaret Knox who allowed me to include her father's inspirational painting *Mount Lefroy*, Adam Tegetmeier who permitted the inclusion of *Boy About to Climb Tree*, and to Thomas Rockwell and the Rockwell Family who allowed reproduction of the detail from *Freedom to Worship*. To the numerous draft readers who provided feedback and encouragement, I am aware of and grateful to each of you. And that includes Dr. John Thie, Dr. Leora Kuttner and Ginger Covalt. To the dear Jewel Compton. To the late Jacquie Osborne who read this manuscript and offered rich feedback despite her failing eyesight, and who told me that dying people don't write books. To Catherine Bennett who got the many permissions off to a rolling start. To Timothy Farrell at RH for being ever efficient. To Patrick Turner who phoned to keep the melodrama in check. To David Noble and Beth Morrison at the BCCA Library. To Anne Syme for her tiny but sharp edits. To Kent Bodell who can (and does) do anything that's required to help. To my niece Alison Edwards and nephews Jason Edwards, Ted Bodell and Tim Bodell who jumped in at tricky spots when I was unwell. To Tom Holmes who always gives me run of his home, his wife and his life. To my youngest nephew Alex Holmes the inventor-writer who never fails to send me green healing energy when it is needed. To Mary in Nova Scotia, her late husband Herb and the Fleury Family for the many prayers. To Anne Gurney. To Evelyn Lau for her good offices. To Paul & Audrey Grescoe. To Michael McCarthy and Gary Tagalog. To Pearl Lemert. To Marcia and Donna Moroz. To Jeanne Ibsen. To Deborah DiGregorio. To Daphne Wilson and Laura. To Dr. Camille Torbey for his friendship. To Linda Hoeppner whose first baby I missed. To Ms. Ronnie Dunne (nee Radcliffe) in Scotland who has always supported me and Glenys Jones in Wales. To Paul Leo and Leigh Shelley who work too hard—thankfully. To St. Therese and the many people who remembered me in kind ways when I was unwell...Thank You.

PERMISSIONS

The author is grateful to the following individuals, organizations, and companies for offering permission to include their works in creation of this book.

The quote on page 23 by Victor Frankl is from *Man's Search for Meaning,* published by Beacon Press.

The excerpt on page 169 by Allan Fotheringham first appeared in *Maclean's,* September 14, 1998. Reprinted by permission of Allan Fotheringham.

The anonymous quotes on pages 269 and 397 were compiled by Ernie Zelinski in *Off the Wall: Graffiti for the Soul,* published by Firefly Books.

The quote on page 321 by David Kessler is from *The Rights of the Dying,* published by HarperCollins Publishers, Inc. ©1997 by David Kessler.

Grateful acknowledgment is made to the following for permission to reprint previously published material:

Bereavement Publishing, Inc.: Excerpt from "The Elephant in the Room" by Terry Kettering. Reprinted by permission of Bereavement Publishing, Inc., 5125 North Union Blvd., Suite 4, Colorado Springs, CO 80918

Leo F. Buscaglia, Inc.: Excerpt from *The Fall of Freddie the Leaf*. Published in the United States by Henry Holt and Co. Reprinted by permission of Leo F. Buscaglia, Inc., P.O. Box 599, Glenbrook, Nevada 89413.

HarperCollins Publishers, Inc.: "Snowball" from *Falling Up* by Shel Silverstein. ©1996 by Shel Silverstein. Reprinted by permission of HarperCollins Publishers, Inc.

Houghton Mifflin Company: Three lines from "Dire Cure" from *After All: Last Poems by William Matthews*. ©1998 by the Estate of William Matthews. Reprinted by permission of Houghton Mifflin Company.

Little, Brown and Company: Excerpt from "City Greenery" from *Everyone but Me and Thee* by Ogden Nash. ©1962 by Ogden Nash. Copyright renewed 1986 by Frances Nash, Isabel Nash Eberstadt, and Liness Nash Smith. Reprinted by permission of Little, Brown and Company (Inc.)

Random House, Inc.: Six lines from "I'm Not Going to Get Up Today" by Dr. Seuss.™ and ©1987 by Dr. Seuss Enterprises, L.P. Reprinted by permission of Random House, Inc.

Charles C. Thomas, Publisher: Excerpt from *Communication with the Fatally Ill* by Dr. Adriaan Verwoerdt, pg. 83. Reprinted courtesy of Charles C. Thomas, Publisher, Springfield, Illinois.

Warner Bros. Publications: Excerpt from "Young At Heart" by Carolyn Leigh and Johnny Richards. ©1954 by Cherio Corporation. Copyright renewed, assigned to Carolyn Leigh and Cherio Corporation. All rights reserved. Used by permission of Warner Bros. Publications U.S. Inc., Miami, Florida 33014.

THE AUTHOR

Arlene Cotter is a graphic designer and writer
living in Vancouver, British Columbia.
Diagnosed with acute non-Hodgkin's lymphoma
in January 1995, she has experienced
treatment, remission, and recurrence.

Arlene now considers herself a survivor
of cancer and lives a normal life.

arlene@peace

— THE AUTHOR'S PROPOSED EPITAPH —